Perioperative Nursing

Edited by

Linda Shields PhD FRCNA
National Health and Medical Research
    Council of Australia
Public Health Postdoctoral Research
    Fellow
Mater Children's Hospital
Brisbane,
Australia

Helen Werder MHS (Health
Services Management) MN, RM, RN
Nursing Practice Co-ordinator
Operating Theatres
Princess Alexandra Hospital
Buranda
Australia

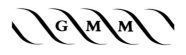

GMM

London ◆ San Francisco

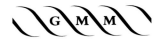

© 2002

Greenwich Medical Media
137 Euston Road
London
NW11 2AA

870 Market Street, Ste 720
San Francisco
CA 94109, USA

ISBN 1–84110–083–8

First published 2002

A catalogue record for this book is available from the British Library.

Visit our website at:
www.greenwich-medical.co.uk

Distributed worldwide by Plymbridge Distributors Ltd and in the
USA by Jamco Distribution

Typeset by Saxon Graphics Ltd, Derby
Printed by Hong Kong Graphics & Printing Ltd, China

Contents

Patient perspectives

Contributors

Maria Anderson
RN, ODP
Clinical Nurse, Operating Theatres, Mater Children's Hospital, Brisbane, Queensland, Australia

Annabel Herron
RN, BN, Cert Perioperative Nursing
Surgical Clinical Support and Product Specialist Device Technologies, Australia

Amanda Silvey
RN, RM
Clinical Midwife Educator, Women's Health Service, Capital and Coast Health; and Clinical Lecturer, Obstetrics and Gynaecology Department, Wellington School of Medicine, Wellington, New Zealand

Linda Shields
PhD, FRCNA
National Health and Medical Research Council of Australia Public Health Research Fellow, Mater Children's Hospital, Brisbane; Adjunct Senior Lecturer, Department of Paediatrics and Child Health, University of Queensland, Brisbane, Australia; Visiting Fellow, School of Caring Sciences, Örebro University, Örebro, Sweden; Visiting Honorary Research Associate, School of Nursing Practice and Midwifery, University of Northumbria at Newcastle, Newcastle-upon-Tyne, UK; and Honorary Fellow, School of Nursing, Queensland University of Technology, Brisbane, Australia

Ann Tanner
RN, MA (Health Science)
Registered Nurse, Operating Theatres, Mater Children's Hospital, Brisbane, Queensland, Australia

Andrea M. Thompson
RN, BN, Anaesthetic Certificate
Clinical Nurse, Operating Theatres, Princess Alexandra Hospital, Brisbane, Queensland, Australia

Lee-Anne Waterman
RN, RM
Registered Nurse, Operating Theatres, Mater Children's Hospital, Brisbane, Queensland, Australia

Helen Werder
RN, RM, MN, MHS (Health Services Management)
Nursing Practice Co-ordinator, Operating Theatres, Princess Alexandra Hospital, Brisbane, Queensland, Australia

Preface

The perioperative area of nursing is exciting, ever changing, always developing. Technology, drugs, anaesthetics and operating procedures change, but ultimately the care of the patient changes little. Nurses who work in perioperative nursing evolve their work practices to keep pace with developments whilst retaining their basic love of caring for people. They are prepared to advocate for their patients in ways that are often more difficult and very different to those encountered on the general wards of a hospital or in the community setting.

This book is written for the beginning practitioner in the operating room, someone who has completed a university degree in nursing or its equivalent but who is a novice in perioperative nursing. Its aim is to provide easy-to-read and easy-to-find information about procedures, conditions and care that the novice to the area may not have encountered before or with which he/she may have had only a passing experience. There are many figures, tables and boxes of information to make gleaning information easy, and to provide interesting background to the text.

The authors are experienced perioperative nurses who have worked in the field for many years. Some are subspecialists in fields such as perioperative care specialists, postanaesthetic care nursing, anaesthetic care nursing or are paediatric perioperative care specialists. Others are clinical educators, or hold combined roles of clinician and educator, clinician and researcher, and clinician and manager. A large section of the book is dedicated to addressing the much-neglected field of paediatric perioperative nursing and also included is a chapter on perioperative midwifery/obstetrics.

While the authors are from the Antipodes, care has been taken to ensure that the content is relevant internationally. References to current research in all areas have been used extensively to broaden and support the knowledge of the authors. This makes the book useful not only for nurses, but also for medical students and others who come to work in the perioperative environment. A full reference list is provided at the end of each chapter. Photographs have been used throughout, most taken by the authors, others taken from accredited hospital libraries' collections.

Because the book is aimed at qualified nurses, every person who reads it will have a basic knowledge of anatomy. However, some chapters do contain drawings and basic explanations of anatomy. We thought it important to include these diagrams and explanations as an *aide-mémoire* so the reader does not continually have to refer to another book while reading this one. There is some repetition between the adult and paediatric sections although paediatric procedures often differ from adult procedures; so, for example, tonsillectomy is described twice, from different perspectives. We had some discussion about the placement of various chapters and sections of chapters. Did anaesthesia in children relate best to Chapter 7 (Anaesthesia) or was it best placed in Chapter 10 (Operative procedures on children)? We opted for the latter, as we felt that if one was reading about operations on children, one would want to access information on paediatric anaesthesia easily. This has occurred several times throughout the book.

The first section contains information about the culture of the operating theatres and its development, the roles of nurses in the perioperative area; legal and ethical considerations; psychosocial perioperative care; and preoperative care. The second section covers basic operating theatre principles; infection control; instruments; safety for both patients and staff; patient positioning and skin preparation. Section 3 contains comprehensive, basic information on operating procedures in adults, anaesthesia and perioperative care of the elderly.

Section 4 is all about children, including the role of parents and the need for a different perspective from an adult viewpoint when nursing children in a perioperative environment, while the final section is about perioperative midwifery care.

The book will provide an easy reference for those who want to look something up, as well as detailed information for the beginning practitioner who is going to work in the perioperative area, whether with adults or children.

All information contained in this book is correct and up to date to the best of our knowledge at the time of writing.

Linda Shields
Helen Werder

Acknowledgements

Many people have helped with this book, by giving advice, checking information, proofreading, re-reading, finding references and photographs, and giving support to us all. We thank the following people in particular, and all those who have helped in any way.

In Brisbane, Queensland, Australia:

At the Mater Misericordiae Hospitals:

Staff of The University of Queensland / Mater McAuley Medical Library,

Staff of the Medical Graphics Department, Mater Education Centre,

Ms Talitha Giddings-Richardson, Indooroopilly, and Ms Karen Richardson, Operating Theatres, Mater Children's Hospital,

Ms Margaret Fletcher, Clinical Nurse Consultant, Operating Theatres, Mater Children's Hospital,

Mr Justin Sharp, Pattison & Barry Solicitors,

Ms Carol Cameron, Clinical Nurse Consultant Infection Control,

Ms Elaine Forster, Clinical Nurse Consultant CSSD,

Ms Beth Burt, Nurse Practice Co-ordinator, Mater Mothers' Hospital,

Sister Josephine Shannon RSM, Archive and Heritage Centre,

Dr Peter Scally, Radiology Department,

Dr Ben Panizza,

At Princess Alexandra Hospital:

Ms Pamela Cummings, Clinical Nurse (Ophthalmology),

Ms Ros Taylor, Clinical Nurse (Gynaecology, Urology),

Ms Jane Gralton, Clinical Nurse (Neurosurgery),

Ms Julia Bucholz-Derrick, Registered Nurse,

Ms Audrey Hamilton, Clinical Nurse (Orthopaedics),

Ms Gillian Lewis, Clinical Nurse (Cardiac Surgery),

Ms Nicki Marr, Registered Nurse,

Ms Chai Tan, Registered Nurse,

Ms Jodie Sisson, Clinical Nurse (ENT, Plastics, Facio-Maxillary),

Ms Lisa Poncini, Registered Nurse,

Ms Jeanne Fremont, Clinical Nurse (Vascular).

Ms Barbara Bryan, Postgraduate Student, Department of Paediatrics & Child Health, University of Queensland,

Mr Terry Ide, Valleylab Division, Tyco Healthcare,

Mr Peter Brinkman, Assistant Director of Nursing, Logan Hospital,

Mr Allan Shields, Moorooka, Queensland, for patience, time and tolerance.

Mrs Judith Hunter MBE, University of Northumbria, Newcastle-upon-Tyne, England, for the initial push to begin this book.

We especially thank Dr Jonathon Gregory of Greenwich Medical Media who encouraged, cajoled and at times bullied us into producing this book. It has been very rewarding and much fun working with him.

Dr Linda Shields is supported by a National Health and Medical Research Council of Australia Public Health Postdoctoral Fellowship Number 997096.

Abbreviations

APL	adjustable pressure limit
ARDS	adult respiratory distress syndrome
ASA	American Society of Anaesthetists
BSE	bovine spongiform encephalopathy
C/S	Caesarean section
CAT scan	computerised axial tomography scan
cm	centimetres
CJD	Creutzfeldt—Jakob disease
CNS	central nervous system
CO_2	carbon dioxide
CSF	cerebrospinal fluid
D&C	dilatation and curettage
DVT	deep vein thrombosis
ECG	electrocardiograph
ECT	electroconvulsive therapy
EEG	electroencephalogram
EMLA™	cream used for topical local anaesthesia
ENT	ear, nose and throat
ETT	endotracheal tube
EUA	examination under anaesthetic
FBC	full blood count
FCC	family-centred care
FESS	functional endoscopic sinus surgery
FFP	fresh frozen plasma
FHR	foetal heart rate
GA	general anaesthetic
ICU	Intensive Care Unit
IM	intramuscular
IV	intravenous
L	litre
LA	local anaesthetic
LMA	laryngeal mask airway
MAC	minimum alveoli concentration (of an anaesthetic gas)
MIS	minimally invasive surgery
ml	millilitres
MRI scan	magnetic resonance imaging scan
NEC	necrotising enterocolitis
NIBP	non-invasive blood pressure monitoring
NVD	normal vaginal delivery
O_2	oxygen
OA	oesophageal atresia
OSA	obstructive sleep apnoea
PACU	Post-Anaesthesia Care Unit
PEEP	positive end-expiratory pressure
PORP	partial ossicular replacement prosthesis
PPACU	Paediatric Post-Anaesthesia Care Unit
PPI	parent present induction (of anaesthesia)
PROM	premature rupture of membranes
RN	registered nurse
SC	subcutaneous
SMR	submucosal resection of the nasal septum
TIVA	total intravenous anaesthesia
TOF	tracheoesophageal fistula
TORP	total ossicular replacement prosthesis
TURP	transurethral resection of the prostate gland
™	registered trademark
UPJ	ureteropelvic junction obstruction
UPPP	uvulopalatopharyngoplasty

Basic principles of perioperative care

1 | Nursing perspectives

Ann Tanner and Maria Anderson

CULTURE OF THE OPERATING ROOM/THEATRE

Ann Tanner

The culture of operating rooms is unique. The operating room (OR) or operating theatre is a complex system that combines personnel, technology, patients and pharmacodynamics in a physical environment coordinated to yield specific patient outcomes.[1] Within the culture of the OR, there is a shift in workplace relations, with interactions between peers rather than with the public. There can be a drama of personalities. This is as much from working in a confined environment as it is from the occurrence of regular, tense episodes during surgery. The theatre nurse's working role has been removed from public scrutiny compared with the nurse working on the wards who is effectively on show to the public and has a public face to maintain. There is a certain comfort in remaining 'invisible' (Fig. 1.1). However, that invisibility can undermine the perioperative nurse's contribution to healthcare and devalue the need for an emphasis on education, counselling, coordination of care and resource management which is inherent in most nursing roles.[2]

The perceived invisibility becomes an issue when health economics and cutbacks in funding impact upon the OR. Many nurses are unprepared for the political manoeuvring and power politics that occur in every institution and this is particularly true in the OR where the unit can remain behind its double doors while the rest of the hospital adapts to economic realities.[3] The perioperative nurse's role in the OR is of a more technical nature than the role experienced by nurses on the wards. Within that

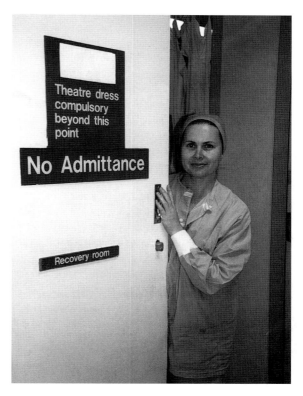

Fig. 1.1 Behind the scenes. Invisibility can undermine the perioperative nurse's contribution to healthcare and devalue the need for an emphasis on education, counselling, coordination of care and resource management

technical function they have a responsibility and accountability for performance of a specialised role, which includes instrument and swab counts, maintenance of aseptic technique, correct use of equipment such as diathermy, endoscopes and lasers, and appropriate patient positioning. There tends to be a well-defined hierarchy amongst nursing staff, dependent upon years of experience and length of stay in that particular area, and the hierarchy is seen also amongst the surgeons and anaesthetists who may prefer working with well-known staff members rather than less experienced nurses.

The culture within the OR can be defined as the sharing of knowledge and experience among nurses.[1] For many perioperative nurses, this sharing of knowledge comes in the form of stories and anecdotes about how they dealt with varying intense theatre experiences. Such stories allow cultural values to be passed on and differing perspectives to be expressed.[2] For many new staff, such anecdotes can form an effective means of learning protocols and procedures. Stories also provide a platform upon which senior nursing staff can express their knowledge and ideas.

Owing to the unpredictable and often hectic environment of the OR, it is essential to maintain a good skill mix amongst staff on each shift with the beginning OR nursing practitioner allocated with senior staff. Some shifts have emergency cases that have priority over elective cases. Nurses who work quickly and efficiently, anticipate problems, plan ahead and interact well within a team are those who progress well in such an environment. It is better to be over prepared in theatre for a case than not prepared at all.

Professionalism within the OR – team focus and the lines of communication

Nurses on the wards who wear uniforms and deal with senior doctors who present in expensive suits can experience barriers in communication which highlight the ascendancy of a medical hierarchy. There is a sense of camaraderie in the OR that begins, perhaps, with the enforced theatre apparel. All staff regardless of position wear the same nondescript loose cotton outfits effectively breaking down potential barriers to communication (Fig. 1.2). However, there can be a conflict between the camaraderie and the lines of power. The hierarchy of power relationships within and between professionals can directly impact on the perioperative nurse. Patient safety and optimal patient outcomes are at issue and it is important for the perioperative nurse to remain focused on patient outcome. To function effectively in the perioperative setting, OR nurses need patience, knowledge and skill in problem-solving techniques, conflict resolution and communication techniques. When healthcare employees cannot manage conflict, friction develops and productivity suffers.[4]

A striking aspect of communication within the OR is the amount of non-verbal cues that occur (Fig. 1.3). Once a nurse is scrubbed or scouting, a surgical mask inhibits much communication. Many hand gestures, signals and other non-verbal means of communication are used during an operation. In some instances, particularly during tense episodes during surgery, it may not be appropriate to interrupt or distract the surgeon. The scrub nurse and scout nurse often resort to eye and hand gestures to communicate between themselves and with others. This silent miming can be quite amusing, but it can take some time to learn for the beginning practitioner in the OR.

As in all areas of nursing, dealing with co-workers in a professional manner is important for the perioperative nurse. Registered nurses in the OR need to communicate ideas, information and problems encountered to the patient, their family, the allied medical and nursing staff, and all levels of medical practitioners from junior doctors to consultant surgeons, physicians and anaesthetists. A team approach to patient care is crucial to the smooth running of an OR. Collaborative relationships among OR staff members are powerful predictors of successful patient outcomes.[2] The ability to develop an easy

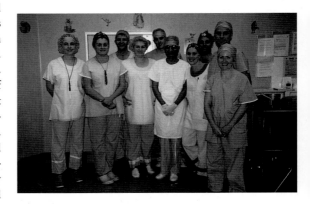

Fig. 1.2 Enforced theatre apparel. This photo includes nurses, anaesthetists, surgeons, anaesthetic technicians and theatre orderlies. Can you spot the professions?

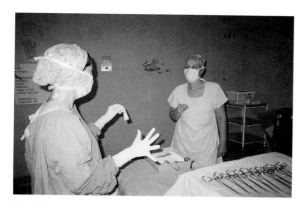

Fig. 1.3 Non-verbal cues. Once a nurse is scrubbed or scouting, a surgical mask inhibits much of the communication. Many hand gestures, signals and other non-verbal means of communication are used during an operation

rapport with the surgeons and anaesthetists as well as the nursing team is essential, but such easy rapport need not disguise the professionalism essential to the OR.

The confines of a health institution, in particular within an OR, can provide an environment where difficult and obstructive personality types thrive. Dealing with these diverse personalities can be extremely stressful. Close teamwork, rapid decisions and confined quarters are all factors that set the stage for conflict in the OR. Conflict occurs when actual or perceived differences exist or when there is a lack of clarity between one or more parties about task accomplishment.[4] The definition of conflict in this instance refers to incompatibilities of goals, actions and values between two or more people.[5] Assertiveness is the most effective means of dealing with conflict. During difficult procedures, the surgeons may become tense and in some instances become stressed. It is important for nurses to maintain their professionalism, remain focused on the case in hand, be alert to what instruments may be required at the differing stages of the procedure and, most importantly, keep track of swabs and other items entering the incision site. The disruptive effect of professional–professional conflict is important because ultimately it will affect the quality of patient care.[6] Successful communication within the OR involves collaboration and cooperation with other team members including the nursing team, surgeons,

anaesthetists and all other allied departments that contribute towards the smooth running of an OR.

Lines of communication with the public

When interacting with the public, it is essential for the perioperative nurse to present as a self-assured advocate capable of articulating and promoting the public welfare.[2] Many people about to undergo surgery are anxious during such a difficult and stressful time. The perioperative nurse is well placed to allay anxieties in a calm and professional manner. The role of patient advocate is an important part of the perioperative nurse's role and includes ensuring that the patient's dignity, privacy and confidentiality remain undiminished in the OR.

It is important to maintain an open and friendly manner and to communicate effectively in difficult circumstances. The perioperative nurse may be required to care for a diverse cross-section of the community. It is essential to remain non-judgmental and view each individual separately, taking into account their own social, economic and emotional situation. Patients have the right to be treated with skill, consideration and dignity regardless of their age, gender, race, religion, disabilities, health and legal status.[7] To succeed in the OR, the perioperative nurse needs to develop an easy rapport with members of the public and their families, and with the other professionals with whom he/she has to work.

COMPUTING IN THE OR

The world passes through cycles of economic growth and prosperity that are related to the use of certain forms of technology. It is currently passing through a growth stage which is driven by the microprocessor. As with the drivers of previous growth stages, it is creating unprecedented change in the technological, economic, social and philosophical frameworks of society.[8] (p. 746)

To keep abreast with such rapid technological change, the OR is incorporating the use of information technology as a powerful tool in analysis, planning and management.[9] The introduction of computers has brought about a change in the methods of data collection from manually written observations, operation details and reports to a

Nursing perspectives

digital database specific to the OR. Information collected on the database includes the procedure description, time taken for the anaesthetic and procedure; staff members, their designation, task and supervision level; types of anaesthetics used, types of prosthesis used; and a whole range of information pertaining to what occurs within an OR. The information gathered is important as it enables appropriate future scheduling of procedures. It is an aid for the compilation of reports for the parent healthcare organisation, be it government or private, and for any accrediting or funding bodies.[10] The OR data are used to assist in a number of classification systems such as diagnostic-related group (DRG) and become a way of describing patient activity.

Before the use of computers in the OR, all information had to be manually recorded, including the operation record, the count sheet and anaesthetic charts. These were then returned to the patient's chart on leaving the theatre. As a rule, the theatre record of the procedure was kept in a book or file with the recording of the date, patient details, procedural details, times, staff and anaesthetics. An electronic database enables the recording of the same information and more; the operation report can then be printed out and kept in the patient's chart, and information is stored in the OR database.[11] The amount of paperwork filed in the patient's chart may remain the same, but the ability of those with need to access all the data stored in the system is greatly enhanced. Computerised OR records allow for retrospective studies on costs, expenditures, prosthetics, staffing mix and allocations.[12] To access the same information manually would take a great deal more time and is far less efficient, although there is some debate about the validity of some computerised records.[13]

As part of the rapidly changing technology, a new information infrastructure has evolved from the fusion of telecommunication and computer technologies.[14] This fusion incorporates the following components.

- Computer systems.
- Telecommunications equipment and optical fibres.
- Satellites.
- Consumer and professional electronics.
- Robotics and flexible manufacturing systems.

- Electronic networks.
- Information content providers.
- Information technology services.

The fusion of telecommunications and computer technologies has been incorporated into the OR with the use of telemedicine. The advent of fibreoptics communication channels has increased the use of telemedicine. Conferences can be videolinked so that a team of surgeons operating can be filmed live in another part of the world.[15] As a result of these technological advances, the remote-area surgeon or general practitioner (GP) can now be assisted and directed online by the specialists in the field via direct video links.

Nursing responsibilities within the OR in relation to computerisation include a need for an awareness of privacy issues (the computerised record is subject to the same rules and regulations as cover all patient records).[16] Nurses must remain educationally up to date with computer systems used in the OR and take advantage of all opportunities offered for upgrading their knowledge about such a rapidly changing field. Nursing research is one of the fields that will benefit most from computerisation and nurses who can tap into such resources will have a wealth of information to analyse and interpret.

NURSING ROLES, AND CLOTHING IN THE OR

Maria Anderson

The roles of the OR staff within the theatre complex are diverse and given varying titles in different parts of the world. Here are described some of the roles of nurses in the OR, but they often overlap. The policies and procedures formulated for work practice within perioperative areas are guided by appropriate legislation in each country. The guidelines adapted from this legislation are used to help each hospital administration, and therefore each perioperative suite, develop its own policies and procedures that guide particular departments. It is imperative that OR staff are aware of the OR policies and procedures of individual hospitals and governing organisations, and that theatre policies must adhere to the legislation and guidelines laid down for the area. Nurses working in the OR take on roles dictated and controlled by such laws and policies.

In the OR there is a designated person in charge of the theatre who is responsible for the efficient running of the operations, for the instrumentation used and for ensuring the surgeon can complete the operation with maximum safety and efficiency. The scrub nurse and circulator or scout nurse together are responsible for the patients perioperative care, as well as ensuring that all documentation is completed correctly. They are also responsible for ensuring all equipment needed during the operation is available.

CIRCULATOR ROLE

The circulator or scout nurse role has many components. The scout nurse is considered the 'extended arms' of the scrub team on whom they rely to provide for them during the case. The role of the scout nurse may involve some or all of the following:

- Act as an efficient professional team member and patient advocate.
- Protect the patient's dignity and privacy by minimising exposure of the patient, keep staff levels to a minimum in each OR and ensure the unconscious patient is treated with dignity at all times.
- Ensure the theatre is prepared according to surgical list requirements and surgeon preferences.
- Ensure patient safety throughout the perioperative phase.
- Have ready electromechanical medical equipment for intraoperative use and carry out required safety checks.
- Carry out cleaning regimes to reduce bacterial counts and the risk of infection.
- Maintain stock levels, ensuring the minimum stock quantity is held in the theatre.
- Admitting the patient to the OR and confirming the patient's identification is an important role for the scout; he/she should ensure the consent form is checked by the surgeon, the anaesthetist and the scrub nurse to ensure the correct operation to the correct site is being performed.
- Act as chaperone for the patient in the anaesthetic room or in the theatre before and during induction of anaesthesia (equally relevant to the anaesthetic nurse's role).
- Complete perioperative documentation clearly

and legibly.
- Provide gown and gloves for the scrub team.
- Assist in the positioning of the patient for surgery.
- Connect the diathermy, suction equipment, tourniquet, air drills and electronic equipment, and be aware of the safety precautions and required settings involved with all such equipment.
- Turn on the operating lights and adjust them as required by the surgeon.
- Open and deliver the required skin preparation and check that the solution is correct and in date. Take care to avoid spilling the solution as wet drapes contaminate a sterile set up.
- Provide sterile instruments as required, open and deliver packages of drapes, swabs, instruments, scopes and other goods as requested by the scrub nurse. Check the integrity of packaging, expiry dates and sterility marker changes. If the pack or instruments' integrity is compromised, do not proceed with the opening, inform the scrub nurse of the problem and find a replacement pack or instrument.
- Document all items for the count of instruments, swabs, etc.
- Collect drugs used for the procedure. Show them to the scrub nurse and both check the product name, strength and expiry date. The scrub nurse will confirm with the surgeon that it is the drug required. The patient may be sensitive or allergic to certain drugs so check this before surgery and inform the surgical team.
- Undue noise should be avoided within the OR while operations are in progress as it may impair communication between team members and distract the surgeon.
- Keep communication between team members clear and effective (can be challenging when wearing surgical masks).
- Collect, label, register and send pathology specimens.
- Ensure the surgeon's preferred sutures and dressings are available.
- Check for the patient's allergies to surgical tapes and inform the surgical team.
- Assist in transferring the patient from the operating table and from the theatre.
- Help remove soiled waste and instruments.
- Prepare the theatre for the next patient.

SCRUB ROLE

Because all OR staff work as a team, the scrub nurse role encompasses many of the circulator nurse duties. The scrub nurse must perform the following:

- Facilitate effective communication within the team.
- Maintain theatre stock levels.
- Prepare theatre according to surgical list requirements and surgeon preferences.
- Ensure all specialised equipment is available.
- Supervise cleaning regimes.
- Assist in perioperative cleaning regimes with the other members of the team to reduce bacterial counts and the risk of infection.
- Ensure all team members carry out the correct scrubbing and gowning-and-gloving technique.
- Open a prepacked drape/tray pack on the trolley, ensure the contents are all present and that their number and type correspond to the list included in the pack. The instruments should be checked thoroughly, be in good condition and be working. Any discrepancies within the check should be documented by the scout nurse on the check list sheet.
- Ensure all trolleys and/or a Mayo stand are available as required and that they are draped appropriately.
- Receive extra instruments required for the procedure from the circulator. Care should be taken when receiving these additions to avoid contamination.
- Check needles, swabs and instruments for the procedure with the circulator and document them. Adherence should be paid to the local policies and procedures.
- Assist the surgeon with gloving if required and tie the surgeon's gown using a sterile technique.
- Check the surgical consent form of the patient before commencing preparing and draping the unconscious patient.
- Prepare and assemble instruments and equipment required for the procedure within the sterile field.
- Observe the patient's position to ensure no damage will be caused through poor positioning.

- Check that the diathermy plate is applied correctly and that there will not be a risk of pooling of the preparation solution on or around the diathermy plate.
- Assist in preparing and draping the patient ready for surgery.
- Have a working knowledge of correct positioning of trolleys and a Mayo stand to allow optimal access to the surgical field.
- Anticipate the surgeon's requirements by following the progress of the surgery.
- Pass instruments to the surgical team as required.
- Carry out second swab, needle and instrument count before the surgeon closes the operative cavity.
- Pass collected specimen to the circulator nurse stating the name of the specimen.
- Prepare sterile dressings and drains as requested by the surgeon in preparation for the end of the surgery.
- Ensure the patient is cleaned of preparation solution or of any other soiling or staining.
- Ensure the patient is in a comfortable position.
- Keep the patient warm with extra blankets if necessary.
- Assist in the transfer of the patient from the table.
- Assist in removing all the equipment from the theatre.
- Prepare the theatre for the next case.

'The count'

Both the scrub and scout nurses are responsible for ensuring that the count of all instruments, swabs, needles and blades used during the operation is correct. This count should be carried out before the operation, before closure of the body cavity and at the end of the operation (Fig. 1.5). If extra countable items are added during the surgery, they must be recorded on the count sheet. The count is documented as per the policy of each hospital, with all relevant sections completed.

Specimen collection

During the surgical procedure, it may be necessary to accept specimens from the sterile field. Gloves and other protective clothing should be worn and documentation completed once the specimen is in the specimen jar. These should be labelled only when the specimen is inserted to avoid the risk of the wrong patient's specimen being put into the incorrectly labelled specimen jar.

ANAESTHETIC ROLE

The anaesthetic nurse's role changes in different countries and hospitals. In some countries and situations, anaesthetic nurses give the anaesthetic, in others they assist the anaesthetist. In some places, they are replaced by anaesthetic technicians who have basic training in anaesthesia and are there only to assist the anaesthetist. They have little legal responsibility and oftentimes have little contact with the patient. For a full explanation of the anaesthetic nurse's role, see Chapter 7.

RECEPTION ROLE

Often a nurse is in charge of the theatre reception area. A nurse's responsibilities include the following.

- Call for patients to be brought to the OR at the appropriate time to ensure there will be no delays in the surgery list and so that the patient is not kept waiting for lengthy periods once he/she has been received in the OR waiting area.
- Provide a calm, restful area and offer psychological support to patients and their families. Allow patients time to verbalise any concerns and attempt to allay any anxieties.
- Check the patient using the preoperative checklist (see page 21).
- Ensure all relevant patient documentation is available such as charts, X-rays and diagnostic test results.
- Ensure the operation site is checked with the patient and/or family and, if necessary, marked.
- Check the operation consent form is dated and signed, with the procedure written in full, the operative side clearly stated and that the patient has given informed consent.
- Act as patient advocate.
- Maintain patient safety until he/she goes into the theatre by ensuring the patient is not left unattended, is kept warm and is secure on the waiting trolley/bed.

RECOVERY ROLE

The Post-Anaesthetic Care Unit (PACU) or recovery room is one of the places where the patient is most at risk.[17] The recovery nurse's role is an expert role that should not be taken for granted. It requires knowledge, skill and experience to maintain the safety of patients when they need frequent, careful and intensive observations, and care. The following information is a guide to the role of the recovery nurse.

The recovery nurse will prepare the area before receiving patients by checking the following:

- Check the resuscitation trolley and document the check.
- Ensure that rebreathing systems are available with all sizes of masks.
- Check that pulse oximetry monitors are switched on and working if available.
- Check the drug cupboard and restock it if necessary.
- Ensure sharps containers and rubbish receptacles are available.
- Check that suction units are clean, functioning, and have the correct and patent tubing attached.
- Check oxygen supplies are adequate and have masks and tubing attached.
- Ensure intravenous (IV) drip stands and IV pumps are available.
- Check that all emergency call bells are working.

The recovery nurse is then ready to receive the patient.

- Receive handover from the surgical team member and the anaesthetist.
- Assess the patient upon arrival.
- Maintain the patient's airway (position the head to open the airway, give jaw support if necessary, use an airway if required and administer oxygen therapy).
- Check breathing (chest movement, feel for air exchange at the mouth, look for signs of cyanosis and observe oxygen saturation levels on the pulse oximetry monitor if available).
- Make observations of circulation (blood pressure and pulse, circulatory observations on limbs, and check drips and drains).

Nursing perspectives

SMITHTOWN CHILDREN'S
HOSPITAL

----ID-------------------------SEX-----UR NO----
SMITH   M   C111111
JOHN
SMITH ST   DOB   16-1-2000
SMITHTOWN
PH (H) 333 333
CATHOLIC

OPERATION REPORT CONT'D

| THROAT PACK | IN | |
| **1 3 MAR 2001** | OUT | |

(Affix Patient Identification Label Here)

Details of count – items	Before Operation	Added during operation						Total	2nd Count	Additions	Final Count
RAYTEC	10							10	10		10
SPONGES	5							5	5		5
~~PACKS~~ VESSEL LOOPS	2							2	2		2
NEURO PATTIES											
PEANUTS	5							5	5		5
HAEMOSTATS	30							30	30		30
BLADES	1							1	1		1
NEEDLES	2	2						5	5	1	6

SIGNATURES: TO INDICATE CORRECT & FINAL CHECK OF ACCOUNTABLE ITEMS
Scrub Nurse_____ (SHIELDS RN) Surgeon_____
Scout Nurse_____ (SNOW RN)
SIGNATURE TO INDICATE CORRECT FINAL CHECK OF OTHER INSTRUMENTS

For discrepancies in count		X-ray Ordered			Taken		Result	
TORNIQUET	Time UP – Arm	R L		Leg	R L			
	Time DOWN – Arm	R L		Leg	R L			

POST OPERATIVE ORDERS

Post-op Investigations   Nil ☐   X-ray ☐   Laboratory ☐

Drugs as per Medication Chart ☐   I.V. Fluids as per I.V. Therapy Sheet ☐

Routine Observations (specify frequency)

Special Observations

Other Orders   Routine   observations
                    IVT   continue   til   oral   tolerated
                    OPD   (1/52)

                              M.O. Signature: _____

Drains. Tubes				
1.	Removed by Checked by	Date		Time
2.	Removed by Checked by	Date		Time
3.	Removed by Checked by	Date		Time

F086B

OPERATION REPORT CONT.

Fig. 1.4 Sample of a completed count sheet

- Assess pain (use a pain measurement tool), reassure the patient, administer drugs as prescribed and reposition the patient as required to make him/her more comfortable.
- Document the patient's condition and care given.
- Prepare the patient for discharge to the ward.
- Hand over all patient information to the ward staff.
- Wash one's hands before and after carrying out a procedure on a patient to minimise the risk of infection.
- Wash one's hands between patients.

While this is a brief overview of the recovery nurse role, it is important to recognise that they are highly specialised professionals who have a vast knowledge of intercurrent disease and its effect on the surgical patient, and the physical and psychological effects of surgery and anaesthesia.

DRESSING AND CLOTHING

Protocols for clothing in the OR are similar the world over. Protective clothing and equipment is supplied by the theatre units and is worn in adherence to local and national policies/procedures within the health and safety guidelines. All personnel entering the theatre complex beyond the demarcation point (the area considered as the clean area and restricted within the complex) must wear theatre clothing. This is loose fitting, comfortable and made of cotton-based material. There are various designs in trouser suits and dresses.

Loose fitting over-gowns should not be worn as they contribute to infection when they fly open and contaminate sterile fields.

Footwear

Footwear should be of a design defined by local health and safety standards and should be worn within the theatre complex only. OR antistatic shoes and boots are available, and because of health and safety issues, there is a move away from the traditional clogs to a full-fitting shoe.

Headwear

Headwear comes in different styles to accommodate the differing amounts of hair a person may have.

Elastic-edged caps are mostly worn by staff with long hair as hair can be tucked inside the cap. Staff with shorter hair often wear caps that tie at the back, though choice is personal. Headwear is lightweight, disposable and comfortable to wear. Often, hoods are worn in orthopaedic theatres. Colourful caps often with cartoon figures are available for children's theatres. However, the general principles of ensuring all the hair is always tucked inside the cap remains the same.

Jewellery

No jewellery other than a wedding ring, should be worn within the theatre complex, and this is removed before scrubbing.[18]

Surgical masks

Masks currently available are made of a lightweight, splash-resistant material that is cool to wear. Masks are available with antifog visors and it is recommended that if the visor mask is not worn then a pair of safety goggles must be worn to prevent body fluids contaminating the eyes. Masks have a flexible bar across the nose area that is compressed around the bridge of the nose. Masks, when originally introduced, were worn to protect the patient from being contaminated with bacteria from microorganisms residing in the nose or mouth of members of the surgical team. With the advent of diseases such as HIV/AIDS and hepatitis, the mask now protects the team members as much as it protects the patient. Current research indicates that masks become ineffective after just a few minutes.[19]

Gloves

Surgical gloves come in many designs and sizes. It is important to establish your correct glove size before scrubbing (Fig. 1.5). Gloves that are too large will inhibit the sense of touch and cause clumsiness. Gloves that are too tight will pinch the fingers and inhibit blood flow and sensation. Surgical gloves provide the most important preventative barrier to contamination provided their integrity is maintained.[20]

Other protective clothing

- Plastic aprons may be provided for protection in cases where large amounts of fluid are used, e.g. urology with irrigation or abdominal washouts.

Nursing perspectives

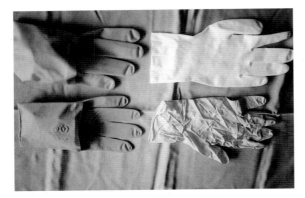

Fig. 1.5 Surgical gloves: sterile surgical gloves are worn during the operation. 1 and 2: Non-sterile latex glove 3: Sterile latex-free glove 4: Sterile latex glove

■ X-rays are often taken in the OR so it is essential to wear protective clothing. Departments provide lead gowns and thyroid protectors.

The use of lasers in the OR is becoming more evident and laser goggles should be provided for all staff within that theatre and a pair should be hung on the outside of the door for anyone wishing to enter the room.

References

1. Reavis C, Sandidge J, Bauer K. Critical thinking's role in perioperative patient safety outcomes. *AORN J* 1998; 68: 758–762, 764, 767–768.
2. Seifert, P. Leading and articulating expertise through stories. *AORN J* 1999; 70: 368–372.
3. Duffy M. Power perceived is power achieved. *AORN J* 1998; 68: 89–92.
4. Pape T. A systems approach to resolving OR conflict. *AORN J* 1999; 69: 551–560.
5. Williams F. *The New Communications*. Belmont: Wadsworth, 1989.
6. Northouse PG, Northouse LL. *Health Communication, A Handbook for Health Professionals*. Norwalk: Appleton & Lange, 1992.
7. *P22 Statement on Patients' Rights and Responsibilities*. Melbourne: Australia New Zealand College of Anaesthetists, 1996. Available from URL: http://www.anzca.edu.au/publications/profdocs/professional/p22_1996.htm
8. Kotler P, Armstrong G, Brown L, Adam S. *Marketing*, 4th ed. Sydney: Prentice Hall, 1998.
9. Gabel R, Kulli J, Lee B, Spratt D, Ward D. *Operating Room Management*. Boston: Butterworth-Heinemann, 1999.
10. McDonald GO, Monosky AD, Montali MA. Surgical informatics is a useful management tool. *Am J Surg* 1997; 174: 291–293.
11. Jones SE. Computers in the operating room: the staff nurse perspective. *Semin Perioper Nurs* 1997; 6: 102–104.
12. Kanich DG, Byrd JR. How to increase efficiency in the operating room. *Surg Clin North Am* 1996; 76: 161–173.
13. Hollenberg JP, Pirraglia PA, Williams-Russo P, Hartman GS, Gold JP, Yao FS, Thomas SJ. Computerized data collection in the operating room during coronary artery bypass surgery: a comparison to the hand-written anesthesia record. *J Cardiothorac Vasc Anesth* 1997; 11: 545–551.
14. Schurr MO, Arezzo A, Buess GF. Robotics and systems technology for advanced endoscopic procedures: experiences in general surgery. *Eur J Cardiothorac Surg*. 1999; 16 (suppl.) 2: S97–105.
15. Lee BR, Bishoff JT, Janetschek G, Bunyaratevej P, Kamolpronwijit W, Cadeddu JA, Ratchanon S, O'Kelley S, Kavoussi LR. A novel method of surgical instruction: international telementoring. *World J Urol* 1998; 16: 367–370.
16. Graveley EA, Brick J. Security and legal issues associated with the computerized patient record. *Semin Perioper Nurs* 1997; 6: 87–93.
17. Hatfield A, Tronson M. *The Complete Recovery Room Book*, 2nd edn. New York: Oxford University Press, 1996.
18. *Standards, Guidelines and Policy Statements*. Sydney: Australian Confederation of Operating Room Nurses, 1998.
19. Belkin NL. The evolution of the surgical mask: filtering efficiency versus effectiveness. *Infect Cont Hosp Epidemiol* 1997; 18: 49–57.
20. Bernthal L. Two gloves or not two gloves, that is the question. *Br J Theatre Nurs* 2000; 10: 102–107.

2 Patient perspectives

Linda Shields and Ann Tanner

PATIENTS' RIGHTS AND THE ETHICS OF PERIOPERATIVE CARE

Linda Shields

There are several aspects of ethical care relevant to the operating room (OR).

CONSENT

All hospitals today have rigid, mandatory policies to be followed when obtaining consent for an operation from a patient. It is important that any patient giving consent for any operative procedure should be fully informed about the reason for the operation, what is going to happen to him/her and the risks involved. By law in many countries it is the duty of the surgeon to explain the procedure and the accompanying risks to the patient,[1] and the anaesthetist has the responsibility to explain the anaesthetic and its implications to the patient before the operation.[2] It is the nurses' responsibility to ensure that the patient has been told and that he/she understands what has been said.[3] This confirmation is done by nurses in the ward preoperatively, and by the nurse who receives the patient in the operating suite. In some hospitals, it is the admitting nurse in the operating suite who must check that the consent form has been signed, in others, the patient cannot leave the ward to be transported to the OR until the consent form is signed. Except in the most extreme emergency situations, no operation can begin without a signed consent form.

If a patient does not seem to understand what is happening to him/her, or if the consent form has not been signed, it is important that the nurse contacts the surgeon and/or anaesthetist. The doctor can then see the patient and ensure they are adequately informed and the consent form has been signed. This must be done before the patient is given any premedication.

How can a nurse check that the patient understands what is going to happen? The best way is to ask the patient outright. However, some patients may say that they understand because they do not want to look foolish or are frightened to say they do not understand. Asking the patient to explain in his/her own words what is going to happen to him/her will show the nurse how much the patient understands.

In the case of children or patients who cannot advocate for themselves, for example the mentally handicapped, the parents and/or family who accompany the patient can give consent.[4] In some hospitals, the right of children to sign consent forms is being recognised, and providing the parent countersigns it, older children are signing their own consent forms. The same principles stand – the child must understand what he/she is signing, must understand what the operative procedure is and what it is for, and must be informed of the risks involved. Any communication with a child has to be age appropriate, and tools such as puppets and calico dolls are good ways to help explain the procedure to a child.

Nurses are ideally placed to tell patients about what the operation will be like and what will happen to them, not only in the operating theatre, but also in the lead up to, and following, the operation. Patients, both adults and children, need to know what to expect. Even for the most informed, intelligent and knowledgeable person of any age, operating theatres and procedures are frightening, anxiety-causing events. The role of the perioperative nurse is to alleviate as much anxiety as possible.

PRIVACY

Patients' privacy can be greatly compromised within the operating theatre. The patient is unconscious and has no control over what is happening. At the same time, his/her body is exposed for the operation and there are numbers of people within the operating theatre at any one time. Theatre suites often have little provision for private conversations, and procedure boards with patients' names and details are often on view to anyone who enters the suite. It is incumbent on all nurses who work in the operating suite to ensure that the patient's privacy is respected at all times. Keep the patient covered as much as possible, restrict visitors to the operating theatres and conduct conversations about private information away from heavy traffic areas. Surgeons often brief the family on completion of a procedure. This is best done in a separate room away from other people.

Children need the same degree of privacy as adults. Just because they are children does not mean they appreciate their bodies exposed. In fact, some children are far more 'body-aware' and modest than many adults are. To expose them unnecessarily is to affront their personal dignity, more so if they are anaesthetised and do not know what is happening to them.

CONFIDENTIALITY

As in all healthcare, the patient undergoing operative and anaesthetic procedures has the right to expect that his/her personal details will be handled in a confidential manner. Charts are treated with the same degree of care as in the wards, not left in places where they can be seen by anybody who does not need access to the information for the care of the patient. When interviewing the patient's family to inform them of the progress of the operation, the surgeon needs a private room or area where he/she can explain confidential information in privacy.

PATIENTS' RIGHTS

Every patient, regardless of age, sex, race, religion or class, has the right to expect to be cared for with dignity and respect. This is as true in the periopera-

tive area as in any other part of a healthcare facility.[5] Extraordinary procedures, an alien environment, odd smells and sounds, people in bizarre clothes, and strange surroundings make up the milieu of the operating suite. Many people think they know what an operating theatre is like from watching television, but often the reality is nothing like their expectations. Some people are terrified at the thought of entering such a place, as it appears totally foreign to them. Any person who comes as a patient (or family) to the operating theatres needs support. Nurses are the best people to give that support because they have the communication skills to make patients less frightened. They also know the value of touch, of reassurance, of being beside the patient, and of talking and explaining what is happening.

Patients have the right to know their safety is assured while in the care of perioperative nurses. This includes emotional and spiritual safety as well as physical. Often patients have operations for life-threatening illnesses and are frightened about what will be found. Sometimes they are having palliative care operations to improve their quality of life and know that their life span will be shortened. Patients often accept the risks of a new procedure in the hope that their life will be improved. Often parents accept these responsibilities for their children. These are frightening situations, and nurses are usually the ones who recognise this and support the patient most effectively.

People from a culture different to the prevailing culture of the hospital have a right to have their particular needs met, including religious and spiritual needs. As an example, Muslims will feel much more comfortable having an operation for removal of a body part if they know they have the choice to decide if that body part (or placenta) will be given to them to dispose of according to their religious laws. Nurses are best situated to find out the wishes of people and to afford them the opportunity of having their wishes respected.

Ethical dilemmas surround contentious issues such as 'do not resuscitate' orders. While advocating for the patient, the nurse must be aware of the laws of the country and act accordingly. However, if a patient has a 'do not resuscitate' order that is legally binding, it is important that the nurse knows this and ensures it is respected.

SELF-DETERMINATION

Patients (or their families) always have choice and it is an important part of OR procedure to ensure those choices are open to the patient. If, at the last minute, a patient decides he/she cannot go through with a procedure, then those wishes must be respected. The good counselling skills of nurses are vital because often a nurse can talk with the patient, help address any queries and issues, and allow the patient to discuss the issues with the appropriate person, be it the surgeon, the anaesthetist or both. Often, these problems are complicated by the fact that the patient has had premedication of some sort and may not be thinking clearly. The nurse assumes the role of patient advocate and coordinates communication for the patient so his/her best interests are assured.

ORGAN PROCUREMENT AND TRANSPLANTATION

One of the most ethically contentious issues faced by the perioperative nurse is the procurement of organs from a brain-dead patient. In many countries today, organ transplantation is an accepted practice. Consequently, the success rate for kidney transplants, for example, is very high. For some other organs, though, the success rates are not so high and the ethics of taking organs for what may be seen as experimental surgery needs to be considered. Cultural values play a part, as some cultures do not sanction organ transplantation.

One of the most distressing situations for a perioperative nurse can be the procurement (commonly called 'harvesting') of organs from a patient who has suffered some insult to the brain and will have no chance of life. Although it sounds easy to rationalise that the giving of the organs will help keep another person alive and that the patient from whom the organs are being taken has no chance of living, organ procurement, particularly from a child or a young person, can cause nurses anguish. This is natural, especially for a beginning perioperative nurse (and not confined to beginners). If one is aware that such issues may arise, then one can at least be prepared. There is nothing wrong with telling the nurse in charge of the shift that one cannot be involved in the procedure.

MEDICAL FUTILITY

Another value conflict with which the perioperative nurse has to deal is medical futility, in other words, is it right to do an operation just because it can be done? While strict codes of ethics govern medical practice, as they do nursing practice, surgeons sometimes fail to see that an operation might be futile to the patient. While it is easy to dictate that nurses must become patient advocates in these situations, in reality it becomes a dilemma when a colleague's work is to be questioned, and nurses may often have to accept what they see as inappropriate activities. In these situations, the nurse can do several things.[6] First, the nurse can assess if the patient (or family) has consented freely to the operation and fully understands what is involved. The rest of the surgical team needs to be consulted and this is usually done in an open meeting. While it may be difficult to stand back and watch what can be seen as a procedure of little benefit performed, nurses must accept the patient's decision to have the operation. If perioperative nurses are aware of their own value systems and can identify and understand fully their own feelings and principles, then they will be better able to deal with problems such as these.

Some healthcare organisations have a qualified ethicist on staff and/or staff counsellors. For any perceived conflict of ethical values, the nurse in charge of the unit can refer nurses in his/her charge to these people.

LEGAL PERSPECTIVES

Perioperative nurses are often at risk of litigation. Although in many cases the hospital takes vicarious liability for the nurse, it is imperative that perioperative nurses hold indemnity insurance to cover them for any potential legal action that may be taken against them. The burgeoning of technologies such as endoscopy and laser, and the increase in responsibility taken by nurses in situations where they become surgeon's assistants has meant a changing of boundaries of what could reasonably be expected of a nurse in the OR. Under the duty of care owed to patients undergoing procedures in the OR, adherence to standards and guidelines for safe practice and detailed, objective documentation ensures that nurses' actions can be seen to be reasonable in a legal action. It is possible that nurses will find themselves involved in lawsuits even though they may not have participated in the incident that caused injury. It is important for nurses to have access to legal counsel to protect their interests. In many countries, professional and industrial bodies provide such coverage, usually, though, only to their members. It is incumbent on nurses to join their organisations and ensure their membership remains current.

A survey of claims against perioperative nurses revealed that the cases for which legal action was taken included retained foreign objects, pressure injuries, medication errors, equipment faults and operations at the wrong site.[7] If nurses ensure their own standards of education and competence are kept up to date, keep abreast of emerging technologies, act in accordance with policies, guidelines and principles in place in their hospital, and document everything carefully, then they will be sure of being able to explain the reasonableness of their actions should it ever be required in a court of law.

EMOTIONAL, SOCIAL AND SPIRITUAL NEEDS OF THE PATIENT

Having an operation can be particularly traumatic for many people and they require special consideration of their emotional and spiritual needs. Patients have the right to know that they are in competent hands and will be treated in a dignified, respectful manner, and that they will be informed of what is going to happen to them in ways they can understand. Perioperative nurses need training in communication skills to ensure the patient understands what they are being told, and patients whose first language is different to the prevailing language of the dominant culture must be provided with translators and written information in their own language.

Many patients find the need to reinforce their spiritual beliefs before impending surgery. Part of good perioperative care is to include the people involved in the patient's spiritual well being as part of the team. They may require a priest, minister of religion or may require counselling from a professional counsellor to help them through this difficult phase. They may require members of their own family to support them, or friends. The nurses' duty is to ascertain the patients' needs and ensure they are satisfactorily met before surgery and in the immediate postoperative period if required. In the case of children, parents should always be allowed to accompany a child to theatre (this is discussed in detail in Chapter 9).

PREOPERATIVE CARE

Ann Tanner

Preparation for operating in a private house
There will be needed: a narrow kitchen table for the operating table (if it is not sufficiently long, place two tables together and tie their legs together firmly to stop them slipping apart), three small tables, and a chair. Choose old furniture. Protect the floor under and around the operating table with rubber or several thicknesses of paper, and cover the rubber with a sheet, securing the sheet at the corners with thumb tacks (Practical Nursing, 1911).[8] (p. 33)

While the OR has progressed from the turn of the century, the basic principles remain the same. Good preoperative care is essential in ensuring that the patient has a sound understanding of what to expect during their stay in hospital. For many patients, it may be their first admission to a hospital and possibly their first experience of an anaesthetic or operation. This can be a nerve-racking experience. Others may have had a previous traumatic experience in hospital, which could make them anxious. It is important for the admitting nurse on the ward and the admitting OR nurse to alleviate such anxieties.

This section examines a number of aspects of admitting a patient to a ward and subsequently to theatre for surgery. It is in the preoperative admission that any perceived complications for surgery must be considered. There are a number of procedures to follow depending on the type of admission, such as day of surgery admission (day surgery), preadmission clinics and emergency admission. It is important to understand the difference between booked elective surgery and emergency admissions, and the difference between a theatre-classified emergency and an acute life-threatening emergency is explained. Procedures involved vary depending on the admis-

**SMITHTOWN CHILDREN'S
HOSPITAL**

PRE-OPERATIVE
CHECK LIST

—ID— —SEX— —UR NO—
SMITH M C111111
JOHN
SMITH ST
SMITHTOWN DOB 16-1-2000
PH (H) 333 333
CATHOLIC

This section is to be completed by RN 30 minutes before transfer to OR	✓ Yes N/A not applicable	Comments
Patient identification band correct and secure	✓	
Presence or absence of allergies documented	✓	Penicillin
Allergy band applied	✓	
Time and nature of last oral intake documented	✓	
Pre-operative medication given and documented	N/A	
Temperature, pulse and respiration documented	✓	
Extra Charts:		
IV, medication, fluid balance, observation sheets	✓	
hospital/private x-rays/laboratory reports	✓	
Pre-operative preparation:		
skin prepared		
bladder emptied		
make-up, nail polish removed		
hairpins, clips or nappy pin removed	✓	
jewellery removed or taped		
presence of loose or damaged teeth noted		
type of prosthesis/implant documented		
Parent/guardian informed of operation:	✓	
Surgical consent form: signed by parent/guardian:		
correct and complete:	✓	
Personal items accompanying child labelled and documented: Trolly hael, dummy ✓		
Where will the parent be while the child is undergoing surgery: Parent's lounge		
Sign and print name of RN completing checklist: (SHIELDS)	Time: 1105 Date: 13.3.01	

This section is to be completed by OR RN:		
Patient identification confirmed	✓	
Identification band correct and secure	✓	
Confirm operation site with parent/guardian or patient record	✓	
Surgical consent form: signed by parent/guardian:	✓	
correct and complete:	✓	
Allergy check confirmed by sighting allergy band/patient chart/ by asking accompanying adult:	✓	Penicillin
X-rays with chart:	✓	
Sign and print name of OR RN: (J. BROWN)	Time: 11:30 Date: 13-3-01	

Fig. 2.1 Completed preoperative check list (paediatric)

sion type but generally include a checklist for preoperative admission, which includes baseline observations, recording the patient's weight, and documentation of surgical and medical history, medications and allergies. The actual preparation for theatre includes fasting, body/site preparation and patient education. This chapter also examines the OR nurse's role in theatre reception, and the protocol to be followed when admitting a patient into the operating suite

ADMISSION BEFORE SURGERY

When the patient arrives in the ward for pre-surgical admission, they will have received information by mail, telephone or from their local doctor about the time of their admission and of the required fasting time. This is usually from midnight the night before morning surgery, and after a light breakfast for afternoon surgery. Most units use a standard checklist for all preoperative admissions (Fig 2.1).

Observation

The first task to ascertain that the patient is fit for theatre is to record a set of baseline observations, including temperature, pulse, respiration and blood pressure. Taking the observations affords the nurse the opportunity to check the patient's skin integrity, particularly around the operating site. Rashes or sores can increase the risk of wound break down and infection following surgery and may result in the operation being cancelled (at the surgeon's discretion). Baseline observations are needed before the anaesthetist's review of the patient. The anaesthetist needs to be made aware of any untoward observations such as pyrexia, hypertension and cardiac arrhythmias to determine if the patient is fit for a general anaesthetic. A fever or an upper respiratory infection may necessitate cancellation of the operation until the patient is well.

Weight

The patient's weight is important for drug calculations and administration. Anaesthetic agents and analgesics are determined on a dose for weight (milligram per kilogram) ratio. The anaesthetist will

ascertain the patient's weight before administering an anaesthetic, so if possible weigh the patient and record it on the anaesthetic chart, the medication chart and the patient's name band. If the patient is bed bound and cannot stand on scales or sit in a weighing chair, the anaesthetist will estimate the weight.

Surgical history

While taking the surgical and medical history is a doctor's responsibility, the OR nurse needs to be aware of anything that can affect the patient's well being. The patient's surgical history is important to ascertain any previous complications with anaesthetics or postoperative complications. He/she may have a history of a reaction to one of the anaesthetic agents. The previous surgery may have included the insertion of a pacemaker or the implantation of some form of prosthesis, e.g. a heart valve replacement, for which the patient may be taking anticoagulation therapy, an important consideration during any surgery. In most instances where the patient has some form of prosthesis or inserted surgical appliance, particularly cardiac, a prophylactic antibiotic may be administered. Some people are more prone to bouts of vomiting and nausea following a general anaesthetic, and if the anaesthetist is aware of this, they may order antiemetic drugs to alleviate the symptoms. Information about all potential problems is important in determining potential postoperative complications likely to arise with each individual undergoing surgery.

Medical history

The patient's medical history may determine risk factors and, if possible, should include a family health history. Whether or not an underlying condition is related to the problem for which the surgery is planned, it still may significantly influence how the surgeon and anaesthetist treat the patient.[9] Frequently encountered conditions include diabetes, coronary heart disease and hypertension. Diabetics are potentially at risk due to the fasting required before theatre and are often given an intravenous infusion to maintain a sufficient level of glucose in their blood. It is important to monitor their blood sugar level (BSL) before, during and following theatre. Patients with coronary heart disease are at risk of suffering a myocardial infarction during a general anaesthetic and may, as an alternative, be given an epidural instead of a general anaesthetic. Patients suffering hypertension may be at risk of a cerebral vascular accident. In modern Western society, the incidence of morbid obesity is increasing and is a causative factor for heart disease and hypertension, and as such becomes a risk factor for anaesthesia. The patient may have a history of bleeding disorders or of venous thrombosis, which puts the patient at risk of a life-threatening pulmonary embolism.

Medications

With any type of medication, it is important to ascertain if the patient has any known allergies and, if so, they must be recorded on the medication sheet, on the patient's chart and clearly marked on the patient's name band. For many patients with pre-existing morbidity, there is a high likelihood that they will be taking some form of medication. These medications may not be compatible with some of the anaesthetic or analgesic agents. Some, such as anticoagulation (aspirin) or anti-inflammatory (steroids) therapies, for example, can affect the success of the operation as anticoagulants increase the risk of intra- and postoperative bleeding,[10] and steroids impair wound healing.[11] All medications need to be recorded, including over-the-counter medications. If known, the patient's compliance with taking medications should also be recorded.[12]

PREPARATION FOR THEATRE

The preoperative patient is often anxious about their surgery and many have little idea of the actual procedure involved. It is important for the admitting nurse to establish the preoperative patient's needs, and the responsibility of the surgeon to adequately inform the patient of the type and extent of surgery required and the associated risks. Preoperative education is of paramount importance, and the admitting nurse can educate the patient on what they can expect when they return from theatre. One of the most frequent concerns of patients about to undergo surgery is the amount of pain they may have. The anaesthetist can

alleviate these anxieties by explaining in detail the type of analgesia they can expect to receive in surgery and postoperatively. The admitting nurse can reiterate this information as well as information about the expected postoperative interventions such as intravenous lines, indwelling catheters, and intravenous or epidural infusions for analgesia. Preoperative education may include the need for antiembolism stockings for those at risk of thrombosis. For some procedures, such as spinal and hip surgery, it may be necessary for the patient to be reviewed and educated by a physiotherapist before surgery to teach them safe methods of turning in bed and for the importance of deep breathing exercises for those who may undergo prolonged bed rest following surgery.

While preparing a child for theatre, family members must be afforded an opportunity to express anxieties and concerns on an individual basis and to determine how they can be most supportive to the child during the perioperative period.[13] The perioperative nurse recognises the importance of input from family members. Communication among the individuals caring for the child is paramount. Established lines of communication permit the efficient and meaningful transfer of information and provide the most efficient means of informing the patient about necessary procedures. Familiarity with OR and day surgery unit policies helps alleviate patient and parent anxieties.

Fasting

For all prebooked elective surgery, it is essential to fast before a general anaesthetic. If the patient has not fasted, there is a risk of vomiting and aspirating food and fluids once the patient is paralysed. The general rule is to fast from all fluids and foods for 6 hours before theatre; children fast for periods relevant to their age. Any drinks or food must be removed from the patient's bedside for the fasting period and a fasting sign placed on the bed to alert others not to provide anything. This signage is particularly important for children who may sometimes wear a 'fasting sticker' or vest, and for adults who cannot communicate. Within the fasting time, the patient may be ordered an oral premedication (usually analgesia or sedation) with a minimal amount of water (20–30 ml).

Body/site preparation

A preoperative shower using antimicrobial skin wash is an important means of reducing surgical site infection. Maintaining skin integrity is a means of reducing the risk of infection. Skin preparation is explained in detail in Chapter 6.

Patients at risk of deep vein thrombosis (DVT) may be required to wear antiembolism support stockings when dressing in their theatre gown. Jewellery must be removed or covered with tape if unable to be removed, as any metal in contact with the patient's skin has the potential to cause burns from the diathermy current. False teeth and dental plates must be removed as they can dislodge during the anaesthetic intubation. Likewise, it is important to be aware of children's loose teeth.

Reception in the operating suite

Entering an OR can be a daunting experience for those about to undergo surgery. Theatre reception is the public face of theatre (Fig 2.2). It is important to introduce yourself and confirm the operative details with the patient using the preoperative checklist.

The patient may be extremely anxious at this stage. Some may claim they do not understand the surgical procedure or the anaesthetic they are about to undergo. In such cases, it is the theatre nurse's responsibility to ensure that the patient can speak with the surgeon or anaesthetist before going into the theatre. The perioperative nurse may be the last healthcare professional a patient encounters before undergoing surgery. Understanding the legal and ethical implications of informed consent enables perioperative nurses not only to act as patient advocate and facilitate solutions to dilemmas, but also to fulfil their legal responsibilities.[14]

When the patient arrives in the theatre reception, a theatre nurse completes the preoperative checklist, which had already been completed once by the nurse on the ward. This checklist includes confirming with the patient that their identification band is correct in all details as to name (including correct spelling) and date of birth, both of which must correlate with the patient's chart. The preoperative check includes verification of any known allergies. Confirm the exact surgery the patient is about to undergo with the patient or his/her family (may include either written

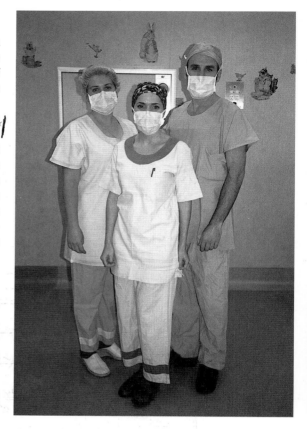

Fig. 2.2 Entering an OR can be a daunting experience for those about to undergo surgery. Remember to remove your mask before entering public areas of theatre as theatre apparel can be threatening in itself.

or verbal consent), including the side of the body it is on and if the patient is well informed and understands the ramifications of the surgery. Confirm when they last took any food or fluids. Relevant X-rays and pathology results must be to hand in the OR. Once these details are established and the correct patient is to undergo the correct procedure, the patient can be accepted into theatre and transferred into the OR.

Day of surgery admission

With advances in surgical expertise and technology, length of hospital stay has been markedly reduced. Procedures that once may have required a 2–3-day hospitalisation are now performed laparoscopically

SMITHTOWN HOSPITAL

DAY SURGERY RECORD

---ID---	SEX---UR NO---
SMITH	M C111111
JOHN	
SMITH ST	DOB 10-8-1950
SMITHTOWN	
PH (H) 333 333	
CATHOLIC	

ADMISSION DATE: 2 April 2001

ADMISSION TIME: 10 am

AFFIX PATIENT IDENTIFICATION LABEL HERE

PRE OPERATIVE CHECKLIST

Identification band	✓	Fasted	✓	Consent	✓	Premedication	✓
X-Ray	✓	Bladder empty (Specify time)	9.45am	Op site prep	✓
Jewellery removed	✓	Make up removed	✓	Nail polish removed	✓	Contact lenses	N/A
Dentures removed	N/A	Theatre clothing	✓	Documentation	✓
Hearing aid removed	N/A				

Loose teeth (Specify) _nil_

Prosthesis (Specify) _N/A_

PRE OPERATIVE NURSING ASSESSMENT

fit + healthy
lives with family
employed full time - gardener
non-smoker

Reason for admission: Surgery - hernia repair

ADVERSE DRUG REACTIONS

Allergic to Penicillin

PREOPERATIVE OBSERVATIONS

DATE	TIME	TEMP	PULSE	RESPS	B.P.	WEIGHT	URINALYSIS	XRAY	ECG	PATH
2.4.01	1000	36⁸	82	16	139/75	70kg	NAD	NAD	NAD	

FASTING FROM: 0600

Pre-Anaesthetic assessment history from questionnaire noted ✓

Remarks

C   MEDICATIONS Nil ✓ Details

D   DRUG REACTIONS: Allergy ✓ Side Effect ☐ Other ☐ Nil ☐ Details _Penicillin rash_

E   ILLNESSES (history or examination): CVS ✓ Resp ✓ CNS ✓ Neuromuscular ✓ Haemo ✓ Renal ✓ GIT ✓ Liver ✓
Endocrine ✓ UGS ✓ Skeletal ✓ Dental ✓ Psychiatric ✓ Obesity ✓ Nil ✓ Details _NAD_

F   ABNORMAL INVESTIGATIONS: ECG ✓ CXR ☐ Hb ✓ WCC ☐ Na ☐ K ☐ Creatinine ☐ Urea ☐ BSL ☐ LFT's ☐
Spirometry ☐ ABG's ☐ Coags ☐ Urinalysis ☐ Others ☐ Nil ✓ Details

G   ASA Rating: 1 ✓ 2 ☐ 3 ☐ 4 ☐ 5 ☐ E ☐   Why?

H   Risk: Good ✓ Fair ☐ Poor ☐ Desperate ☐   I. Technique Suggested: GA ✓ Regional ☐ Infiltration ☐ Sedation ☐

J   COMMENTS

PRE-MED   Signature _____ Simons   Date 2/4/01

DATE ORDERED	DRUG	DOSE	ROUTE	M.O. SIGN	DATE& TIME GIVEN	GIVEN BY	R.N.'S SIGN
2.4.01	Temazepam	10mg	PO	m	2/4/01 0945	J Smart	J Smart
	Ranitidine	150mg	PO	m	2/4/01 0945	J Smart	J Smart

MR074

Fig. 2.3 Completed preoperative check list (adult)

and the patient is discharged either the same day or after a night's stay. Procedures that allow the patient to be discharged on the same day of surgery significantly reduce the cost of healthcare and limit unnecessary bed occupancy. The type of procedures suitable for day surgery must have a minimal risk of postoperative haemorrhage, a minimal risk of postoperative airway compromise and controllable pain that can be managed with oral analgesics at home.[15] To be fit for discharge on the day of surgery, the patient needs to tolerate food and fluids, to have voided postoperatively, and to be relatively free from pain and discomfort. The day-surgery patient must have a responsible adult to transport them home in a suitable vehicle and a responsible person at home for at least the first night after discharge.

Procedures for a day surgery admission include the standard preoperative checklist, including baseline observations, surgical and medical history, allergies, medications, fasting times and an understanding of procedures. Each unit has standard admission times for morning and afternoon theatre lists to ensure enough time for surgical and anaesthetic review before theatre. In some cases, the patients have been surgically reviewed before admission and may have already signed a consent form for surgery. The anaesthetist reviews the patient on the day of surgery to ensure they are fit for an anaesthetic.

Preadmission clinic

Patients sometimes attend a preadmission outpatient clinic or their private doctor's rooms before surgery for the preadmission examination. This provides an alternative to the costs of an overnight admission before theatre. At the preadmission visit, tests and blood cross-matching may be required if the patient is to undergo major surgery. Baseline observations are recorded in the clinic as well as on admission to the ward. Pre- and postoperative education is given at the clinic. Often consent for theatre is signed in the preoperative clinics. The patient's history is recorded, including medications and allergies, surgical and medical history and any complications of previous surgery or anaesthetics. The preadmission clinic provides a non-stressful environment in which questions about surgery can

be clarified. On the day of surgery, there is often less time to alleviate anxieties than there may be in a clinic setting.

Emergency admission

In OR terms, an emergency admission includes any procedure that requires treatment within 12–24 hours. An example could be a fractured limb or abdominal pain with suspected appendicitis. In such cases, there is time for the ward staff to perform the standard preoperative admission, observations, and surgical and family history. Emergency patients will often be admitted to the ward whilst waiting for theatre time to become available. A true emergency such as an acute airway obstruction where an emergency tracheostomy may need to be performed would bypass preadmission checks and come directly into the OR. The patient will arrive directly from the accident and emergency department and routine theatre cases are delayed until the emergency case has been completed. In the case of a multiple trauma (such as a motor vehicle accident), the patient may need to undergo X-rays and computed tomographic (CT) scans before admission to theatre to ascertain the extent of the trauma, particularly in the case of head injury. In these acute emergency admissions, allergies and medical history may be obtained from relatives or friends if time permits.

OR staff will have time to set up a theatre in preparation for the procedures involved, including organising the equipment and instruments required. On some occasions, there is little warning or preparation time, so it is essential to leave all theatres set up to the extent that the bed and anaesthetic machine are in the correct place, that the theatre is properly stocked, and that the oxygen, suction, diathermy and lighting are all functioning and ready for use.

References

1. Breen K, Plueckhahn V, Cordner S. *Ethics, Law and Medical Practice*. St Leonards: Allen & Unwin, 1997.
2. Australia New Zealand College of Anaesthetists. *P22 Statement on Patients' Rights and Responsibilities*. Melbourne: Australia New Zealand College of Anaesthetists, 1996. Available from URL:

http://www.anzca.edu.au/publications/profdocs/professional/p22_1996.htm

3. Murphy EK. Preparation of the patient for the procedure: legal and ethical considerations. In: Phippen ML, Wells MP. *Patient Care during Operative and Invasive Procedures*. Philadelphia: WB Saunders, 2000.

4. Kerridge I, Lowe M, McPhee J. *Ethics and Law for the Health Professions*. Katoomba: Social Science, 1998.

5. *Anon.* Patients more satisfied when informed of their rights. *AORN J* 1999; 70: 107.

6. Schroeter K. Medical futility: interpretation and ethical ramifications for the perioperative nurse. *Semin Perioper Nurs* 1997; 6: 138–141.

7. Murphy EK. Types of legal claims brought against perioperative nurses. *AORN J* 1997; 65: 972–973.

8. Pope A, Maxwell A eds. *Practical Nursing*. New York: GP Putnam, 1911; cited in Murphy E. Perioperative nursing in the early 1900s *AORN J* 1999; 70: 33.

9. American Academy of Pediatrics. Evaluation and preparation of pediatric patients undergoing anesthesia. *Pediatrics* 1996; 98: 502–508.

10. MIMS Pharmaceutical Database. *Aspirin.* Available from URL: http://intranet.mater.org.au/mims/DSPPROD.ASP?ACT=DSPC&MRN=342&KEY=197

11. MIMS Pharmaceutical Database. Prednisone. Available from URL: www.mims/DSPPROD.ASP?ACT=DSPC&MRN=688&KEY=401

12. Martinelli AM. Administering drugs and solutions. In: Phippen ML, Wells MP. *Patient Care during Operative and Invasive Procedures*. Philadelphia: WB Saunders, 2000.

13. Kristensson-Hallstrom I. Parental participation in pediatric surgical care. *AORN J* 2000; 71: 1021–1029.

14. Pryor F. Key concepts in informed consent for perioperative nurses. *AORN J* 1997; 65: 1105–1110.

15. Australia New Zealand College of Anaesthetists. *Review PS15* Recommendations for the Perioperative Care of Patients Selected for Day Care Surgery. Australian and New Zealand College of Anaesthetists. Melbourne, 2000. Available from URL: http://www.anzca.edu.au/publications/profdocs/profstandards/ps15_2000.htm

Patient perspectives

Environmental safety | 2

3 | Infection control

Helen Werder, Maria Anderson, Annabel Herron and Linda Shields

TRAFFIC PATTERNS WITHIN THE PERIOPERATIVE AREA

Helen Werder

Traffic patterns within the perioperative area will reflect variations in practice settings and/or clinical situations and the multiple different settings within which perioperative nurses practise. Included in these practice settings may be the traditional operating theatres, day surgery units, endoscopy units, radiology units, and cardiac catheterisation units and any other areas where surgery is performed.[1]

Care of the perioperative patient requires the movement of patients, personnel and equipment within and through the perioperative unit. The controlling and planning of these movements with designated traffic patterns based on the design of the unit assists in the containment of contamination. Traffic patterns direct movement into and out of the surgical unit and movement within the unit. Facilitation of the flow of traffic and the definition of areas within the unit should be directed by signage that indicates the appropriate environmental control and surgical attire required.

The perioperative unit should be designated into three areas defined by the physical activities performed in each area.

An unrestricted area includes the central control point where monitoring of the entrance of patients, personnel and materials into the unit is established and where traffic is not limited and street clothing may be worn. Communication between personnel within the unit and the external health facility environment is transacted within this area.

A semirestricted area includes the transition areas for the processing of supplies into the unit, the peripheral support areas for the storage of clean and sterile instruments, the corridors to the restricted areas of the perioperative unit and where prepared day-surgery patients await transfer. Personnel within this area are required to wear theatre attire and patients are required to wear gowns and hair covering.

The restricted area is where surgical procedures are performed and the sterile preparation areas and scrub areas are located. Within these areas, surgical attire as designated by the policies of the facility is required to be worn at all times.[1,2]

The traffic flow should progress from unrestricted areas to either semirestricted or restricted areas and the transition zones dividing each area from the next should not be transgressed without adhering to the appropriate dress codes.

Traffic flow within the surgical area should be kept to a minimum. This can be enhanced by several simple measures.

- Careful planning of the perioperative episode keeps the traffic into and out of the operating room (OR) for extra supplies to a minimum, thus reducing the amount of airborne contamination caused by increased movement.
- The decreased opening and closing of doors diminishes the mixing of OR air with corridor air and therefore maintains the positive air pressure within the immediate environment, which lowers bacterial counts.
- Decreased movement, talking and the number of personnel present during surgery keeps air currents to a minimum, thus decreasing the amount of contaminated particles shed from patients, personnel and drapes. Shedding increases with activity and accelerates the risk of higher bacterial counts.

- Clean and sterile supplies and equipment movement should be separated as much as possible from contaminated supplies, equipment and waste by space, time or traffic patterns.[1]
- Sterile supplies and instruments for surgical cases should be transported to the OR in covered trolleys, and traversing unrestricted areas where airborne contaminants and contact may contaminate them should be avoided.
- Supplies and equipment should be removed from external supply containers in the unrestricted area before transfer into the restricted areas.
- Soiled supplies, instruments and equipment should be transported for decontamination and disposal along routes that exit the restricted areas as quickly as possible to avoid cross-contamination of clean supplies and equipment.

Traffic patterns may be affected by current evidence-based practice research, by construction, renovation and maintenance, and should therefore be reviewed frequently to improve the guidelines for policies and procedures and to improve quality assessment of practice.

SURGICAL SCRUB

Maria Anderson

The risk of infection was recognised in the 14th century when the Venetians quarantined themselves from the Black Death. In 1807, Giuseppe Alessandro Gianni stopped an epidemic of typhus by making carers wash their hands in diluted acetic acid and disinfecting the nursing area;[3] and Ignaz Semmelweiss in 1861 published a paper that showed that he had reduced the deaths of women from puerperal fever by making doctors wash their hands.[4]

The surgical scrub reduces the bacteria count on the skin and the risk of infection to the patient,[5,6] and the formal surgical scrub has been the subject of much research.[5-7] Views about how long a surgical scrub should take vary widely,[7] with times ranging from 2 to 5 minutes. Nurses should follow guidelines provided by the hospital in which they work, or by the policies, procedures and standards written by relevant professional bodies. The scrub technique can be broken down into six separate elements.

- Duration and sequence of the scrub: adhere to local guidelines from 2 to 5 minutes.
- Scrub solutions: hospitals provide several different solutions that can include iodine- or chlorhexidine-based solutions. Some are drying and irritate the skin and the nurse can usually choose from the solutions provided.
- When and how to use scrub brushes: scrub brushes are necessary to clean the subungual area. Brushes can be disposable or reusable and when used at the start of the hand-washing technique they should be used on the subungual area only and then discarded. Some controversy surrounds the use of brushes, with many advocating that they should not be used,[8] while others have found that new chemical scrub compounds obviate the need for brushes.[9]
- Position of the hands during scrub: keep the hands above the elbows at all times to prevent contamination from water running from the unclean elbow down the arm.
- Rinse technique: rinse from the finger tips to the elbows with the hands at a level above the elbows at all times to prevent contamination from water from the unclean elbow running down the arm.
- Drying technique: wipe the hands and arms with a sterile wipe from the fingertips to the elbows using a twisting action of the towel rather than an up and down action. Then discard the towel once the elbow has been reached. The effective drying of hands plays a significant part in the reduction of the bacterial count on the hands.

All these factors influence the effectiveness of a surgical scrub. The surgical scrub may seem a minor step particularly when overshadowed by impressive surgical technology. However, all this may fail if the surgical scrub does not prevent the transmission of bacteria.

GOWNING AND GLOVING

Gowning

Sterile gowns and surgical gloves are packed in a way that allows them to be handled without touching the outside of the item. The scout nurse should open the gown ready for the scrub nurse, whose hands should be dried thoroughly before picking up the gown. The scrub nurse picks the gown up by the inside of the shoulders and holds it to allow it to unfold. It is then opened to expose the inside of the sleeves. Both hands are pushed into the sleeves simultaneously, but no effort made to adjust the gown. The scout/circulating nurse will adjust the gown onto the scrub nurse's shoulders by holding onto the top inside ties. The scrub nurse's hands must not protrude from the end of the gown.

Once the gown is on, the nurse can don gloves.

Gloving

There are two recognised ways of donning sterile gloves.

Closed glove technique

Keep the hands and fingers inside the end of the surgical gown and touch things with the inside fabric of the gown only. Lay the gloves within their packet with their fingers toward you. Pick up the left glove using the right hand and place it on the palm of the left hand with thumbs together. Hold the cuff of the glove between the thumb and the forefinger ensuring they remain within the confines of the gown. Grasp the uppermost cuff with the right thumb and forefinger and flip the glove over the end of the hand. Pull it into place on the hand and over the cuff of the gown. Repeat the same steps for the other hand.

Open glove technique

Hands or fingers should not touch the **outside** of the glove. Open the glove packet out carefully and tip it on to the sterile draped area on the trolley. Pick up the right glove by the left hand holding it at the inside cuff. Push the right hand carefully into the glove while gently pulling back on the cuff. When the hand is inserted into the glove, the cuff is released. Place the fingers of the gloved hand under the cuff of the left glove and gently insert the hand into the glove the same as was done for the right side. Once the fingers are inside the cuff, it should be flicked back over the sleeve of the gown. Place the gloved fingers under the cuff of the right glove and flick this cuff back as before.

SKIN PREPARATION AND DRAPING

Helen Werder

Preoperative skin preparation

Many bacteria are found on the skin, and because the skin cannot be sterilised, it is important to reduce the microbial count to as low as possible to aid in the prevention of wound infections. The skin is divided into two layers: epidermis and dermis. The dermis is a connective tissue layer containing the blood and lymph vessels, sweat and sebaceous glands, nerves, and hair. The epidermis constantly sheds the new cells that replenish the surface every day and contains no blood vessels but has hair shafts, glandular ducts and fine nerves reaching through it to the surface. The bacteria found in the layers of the skin comprise two groups: transient and resident flora. The transient flora usually lie freely on the surface of the skin or are attached by grease or dirt and are removed by mechanical cleansing of the skin. The resident flora adhere to epithelial cells and extend downward toward the glands and hair follicles.

The skin requires thorough preparation at both the pre- and intraoperative phase. The preoperative phase should involve a shower/bath the evening before and again on the morning of surgery with an antimicrobial agent, and in some instances the removal of hair directly involved with the proposed incision site. (This procedure will be dependent on the policy of each hospital, as some only require one shower/bath with the antimicrobial agent. Also, some hospitals require the preoperative shave or clip for hair removal to be performed immediately before or as close as possible to surgery.) If a shave is to be performed, the wet shave method should be utilised as it facilitates hair removal, minimises skin trauma, and prevents dry hair and debris from becoming airborne.[10]

Nursing considerations

- Adequate instructions must be given to the patient in the use and application of the antimicrobial agent.
- The general condition of the patient's skin should be observed for any abnormal conditions that would contraindicate surgery or for any reaction to the antimicrobial solution. Any conditions that

would prevent surgery should be reported to the surgeon.

- Privacy and adequate explanations must be given to the patient when performing the shaving procedure.
- The shaving nurse must have a good knowledge of the proposed shave areas before commencement of the procedure.
- When wet shaving, the antimicrobial agent should be compatible with the antimicrobial agent contained in the skin preparation solution.
- When using a disposable razor, the skin should be held taut and the razor moved in the direction of hair growth.
- When using clippers, the skin should be held taut and the clipper moved in the direction of hair growth.
- When using clippers, use a fresh disposable clipper head for each patient.
- Avoid creating nicks or abrasions in the skin. If this happens, the surgeon should be informed.
- Never shave eyebrows or cut eyelashes unless specifically ordered to by the surgeon.

Intraoperative skin preparation

To avoid postoperative infections resulting from contamination acquired in the OR, the skin at the incision site and in the area surrounding the region of surgery should be prepared using an antimicrobial solution. Surgical infections can be a result of microbial contamination of the wound, the condition of the wound at the end of surgery or patient susceptibility, or a combination of all three.[10] The condition of the wound at the end of surgery will be determined by the actual surgical technique. The perioperative nurse can contribute to the prevention of surgical wound infections by correct preparation of the incision site.

Antimicrobial agents should be selected to be active against both Gram-positive and -negative bacteria. Two generic groups of agents are provided in the povidone/iodine and chlorhexidine gluconate solutions. These solutions are rapid acting, are not dependent on cumulative action, have a broad spectrum of activity in reducing transient/resident flora and inhibit rapid rebound growth of microbes.[10] The contact time of the agent on the skin before surgery is commenced should be based on the documentation provided with the solution.

Skin preparation technique

The instrument and swabs used to apply the antimicrobial solution vary greatly. Basically, they consist of a container to hold the preparation solution, a swab-holding instrument and a swab to absorb the solution.

Regardless of what applicator is used, the principles of performing the aseptic procedure are the same. The preparation begins at the incision site and works outwards to the periphery of the chosen area. The preparation swab should never cover an area already covered with that swab. A fresh preparation-soaked swab should be used for each additional application of the antimicrobial solution. The chosen boundaries of the preparation site should adequately cover the area of the incision and any area in the surrounding surface that may be used for the insertion of drains. The area should have a sufficiently large margin that the sterile drapes are not at the edge of the prepared area. Areas considered dirty or contaminated should be prepared last such as the perineal area, axilla and umbilicus. Cotton-tipped applicators may be used to prepare small confined areas such as the umbilicus.

Nursing considerations

- Nurse should ensure that the patient has no known allergy to the antimicrobial solution.
- Maintain an aseptic technique throughout the procedure.
- Chlorhexidine gluconate solution should not be used for or near the eyes, ears or mouth.
- Care should be taken that pooling of the preparation solution does not occur, especially at the diathermy site or under the patient where chemical burns may result.
- Care should be taken when preparing open wounds or comminuted fractures over which the solution may be poured instead of painted on.
- Avoid going over areas already prepared.
- Discard the swab after use.

Skin preparation area guidelines

Surgical preparation guidelines are illustrated in Figs 3.1 – 3.9 on pp 17–19.

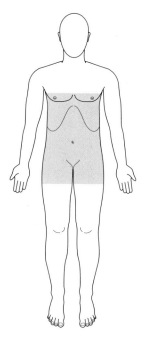

Fig. 3.1 Preparation of site: abdomen

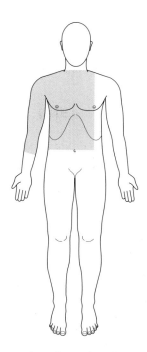

Fig. 3.2 Preparation of site: chest/breast

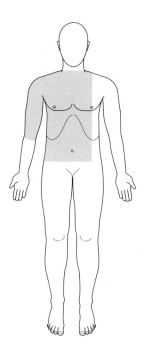

Fig. 3.3a Preparation of site: lateral/thoracotomy

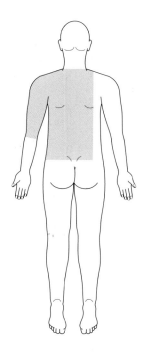

Fig. 3.3b Preparation of site: lateral/thoracotomy

Abdomen

Whilst in a supine position, the area should include from the breastline to the upper third of the thighs, and from the table line on one side to the table line on the opposite side.

Chest/breast

While in an elevated supine, supine or lateral position, the area should include the shoulder, the upper arm to the elbow, the axilla, the chest wall to the table line and to the line of the nipple towards the opposite shoulder and inferiorly to the umbilicus.

Lateral/thoracotomy

The area should include the chest and abdomen from the neck to the iliac crest anteriorly extending over the midline to the nipple line on the opposite side if possible. Posteriorly, the area should include the chest and back from the neck to the iliac crest and extending to the table line if possible.

Rectoperineal/vaginal

In females, the area includes the pubis, vulva, labia, perineum, anus and adjacent areas, including the inner aspects of the upper third of the thighs. In males, the area includes the pubis, genitalia, perineum, anus and adjacent areas, including the inner aspects of the upper third of the thighs.

Abdominal/perineal

This area includes from the breastline to the pubis area and the rectoperineal area as previously described, and from the table line on one side to the table line on the opposite side of the abdominal area.

Knee/lower leg

This area includes the full circumference of the leg for surgery and extends from the upper thigh to the foot. The area may also include preparation of the foot.

Hip/lower extremity

This area includes the abdomen on the affected side, the buttocks to the table line on the opposite side, the groin, the pubis and the circumference of the thigh to include the foot.

Hand and elbow

This area includes all the hand, with particular attention to the spaces between the fingers, to the tourniquet.

DRAPING

Maria Anderson

Sterile drapes have been used for many years to provide a sterile field on which the surgeon can work. Fabric drapes have traditionally been used as they can be washed and sterilised effectively, but in latter years disposable drapes have become more common. The debate about the efficacy of disposable versus reusable drapes centres around the permeability of the material, the cost, the possibility of contamination and the ease of use.[11,12] Draping is known to affect temperature control[10] and gas exchange[13] during surgery. Increasingly, self-adhesive drapes[14] are replacing fabric drapes held in place with towel clips.

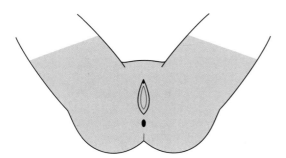

Fig. 3.4 Preparation of site: rectoperitoneal/vaginal

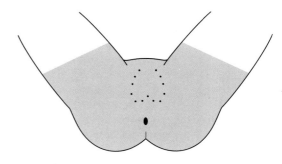

Fig. 3.5a Preparation of site: abdominal/perineal

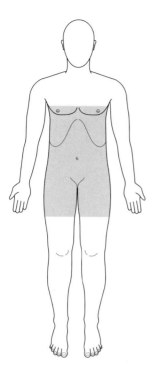

Fig. 3.5b Preparation of site: abdominal/perineal

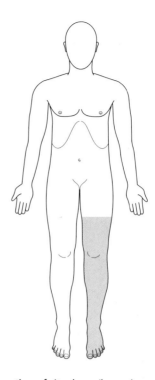

Fig. 3.6 Preparation of site: knee/lower leg

There are various draping procedures relevant to respective operations, and it is beyond the scope of this book to explain them all. They are very well illustrated in Phippen and Wells[15] and Meeker and Rothrock.[2] The basic principles for draping a patient are the following.

- Draping is done according to the policies of respective ORs.
- Draping is done by two people in sterile gowns and gloves.
- Placement of the drapes depends on the procedure to be performed.
- Material should be non-flammable because of the use of diathermy and gases.
- Material must be lint free.
- Any drapes that are moist or have holes may be contaminated and should be discarded.
- Once in place, drapes cannot be repositioned.
- Sterile drapes are placed over the anaesthetic screen that separates the sterile and non-sterile area.

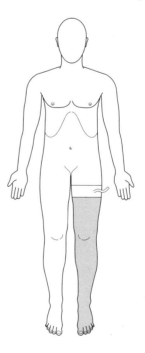

Fig. 3.7 Preparation of site: knee/lower leg

Infection control

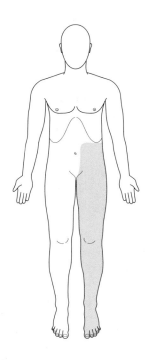

Fig. 3.8 Preparation of site: hip/lower extremity

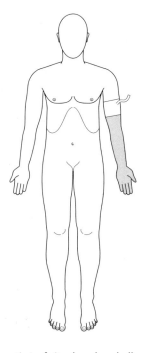

Fig. 3.9 Preparation of site: hand and elbow

■ Sterile, waterproof drapes can be used under drapes to prevent the seeping of moisture, thus contaminating the field from below the drape.

■ If adhesive drapes are used, the patient's skin must be completely dry.

DECONTAMINATION, CLEANING AND MAINTENANCE OF INSTRUMENTS

Helen Werder

The perioperative nurse needs to be aware of the information on the decontamination, cleaning and maintenance of instruments to provide a safe environment for the patient. Instruments used during the surgical procedure should only be used for the specific purpose for which they were designed. This correct usage ensures the continuing effectiveness of the instrument and decreases the likelihood of delays in the surgical procedure and the risk of infection and patient injury.

Intraoperatively, the instruments should be kept free of gross contamination and the lumens kept patent. Instruments contaminated with blood and secretions result in possible corrosion, rusting and pitting when blood and debris are allowed to dry in or on the instrument. Instruments with lumens may become obstructed with debris and organic material, thus hindering the progress of the operation. Instruments should never be allowed to soak in or be cleaned with saline as this increases rusting, pitting and discoloration of the instrument surface. Fine and delicate instruments should be kept separate from heavy instruments to avoid surface damage and distortion of the instrument. Endoscopic telescopes and instruments should be kept as much as possible in containers separate from other instrumentation to avoid damage.

Postoperatively, the instruments should be decontaminated and cleaned as soon as possible to the completion of the surgical procedure. As the presence or otherwise of pathogens at the time of surgery is unknown, this immediate decontamination is necessary for the protection of personnel and the prevention of transmission of these pathogens. The decontamination/cleaning process for surgical instruments should include prerinsing or soaking, washing, rinsing and sterilising. Prolonged soaking is not recommended as extended exposure to detergents and solutions may damage the instrument surfaces. This process should take place in an automated washer steriliser with detergents that are non-corrosive, low sudsing and with a pH close to neutral. Abrasive scouring powders and scouring pads should not be used as they will scratch the finish on the metal, thereby increasing the possibility of corrosion. Instruments should be arranged either in metal trays or suspended on racks so that all surfaces are exposed to the action of the automated cleaner.

Instruments should be prepared in the following ways.

- Box joints should be opened.
- Instruments with removable parts should be disassembled.
- Instruments such as scissors should be opened.
- Heavy instruments should be placed separately.
- Light instruments should be placed on the surface with microsurgical instruments kept in an enclosed but water-penetrable container to avoid loss of small parts.

When the manufacturer recommends natural cleaning or the facility cannot access automated washers, personnel should wear the recommended protective attire and the instruments should be cleaned while submerged in the appropriate detergent and warm water. Submersion will protect personnel from aerosolisation and splashing of infectious material during cleaning. Care should be taken in the manner of cleaning to avoid cuts, sticks and injuries from sharp instruments.

Following initial decontamination, it is recommended that instruments be then processed through an ultrasonic cleaner to remove small particles of debris from the crevices. Instruments should then be rinsed to remove the cleaning solution and small particles of debris. The manufacturer's instructions on the combination of dissimilar metals should be followed as non-compliance will result in ion transfer causing etching and pitting of instrument surfaces. All instruments must be thoroughly dried before sterilisation or storage. Maintenance of instruments commences with an inspection before storage or sterilisation, which should include the following.

- Cleanliness of difficult-to-access joints and lumens.
- Alignment of jaws and teeth.
- Absence of hairline fractures in box joints.
- Sharpness of cutting edges.
- Smoothness and sharpness of instruments such as chisels, gouges and osteotomes.
- Ability of needle holders to hold needles without movement.
- Absence of chips, worn areas and sharp edges from chrome instruments.
- Treatment of stiff instruments with water-soluble lubricant.

All defective instruments should be sent for maintenance, repair or replacement.

Rigid or flexible endoscopes and endoscopic instrumentation should be handled to prevent damage to lenses and fibreoptic components. Endoscopes should be disassembled and thoroughly cleaned with extra attention being paid to channels, crevices, joints, taps and fibreoptic attachment sites. This is best accomplished by gentle rinsing with flushing of channels, then cleaning in an endoscopic processor. After thorough cleaning, it is imperative that all channels and connections are thoroughly rinsed and dried to permit maximum contact with steam sterilisation methods or disinfection with chemical germicides. Where decontamination and disinfection of difficult biopsy forceps and cytology brushes are involved, single-use disposable equipment is more efficient and safer. Before disinfection or sterilisation of endoscopic equipment, insulation on instruments should be visually inspected for cracks or tears and the instrument tested with a laparoscopic insulation testing unit to detect microscopic breaks in the insulation. Endoscopes and instrumentation should be inspected for damage and cleanliness and tested as per the manufacturers' guidelines.

Powered surgical instruments should be decontaminated and cleaned immediately after use to remove organic debris that will hinder the functioning of the equipment and the sterilisation process. Residual organic debris will cause corrosion of the inner working process of some makes of powered surgical instruments. The methods of decontamination should be in keeping with the manufacturers' guidelines and should specifically include the following.

Infection control

- **Non**-immersion of powered surgical instruments and air hoses in water, or solutions in automated or ultrasonic cleaners.
- Inspection of the hoses and cords for damage or wear.
- Attachment of air hoses of powered surgical instruments to the handpiece during cleaning.
- Cleaning with an appropriate detergent.
- Careful removal of organic debris and cleaning of cannulated powered surgical instruments.
- Thorough rinsing and removal of detergent from the powered surgical instrument and the air hose with a damp cloth.
- Drying of the powered surgical instrument and the hose with a lint-free cloth.
- Lubrication of powered surgical instruments and accessories according to the manufacturers' guidelines. Some powered surgical instruments need to be run after lubrication to ensure dispersion of the lubricant within the internal mechanism.

Powered surgical instruments and their hoses and attachments should be inspected and tested before sterilisation to ensure:

- proper seating of the attachments; and
- triggers, handles and key chunks are in good working condition.

Before sterilisation, the powered surgical instrument should be disassembled with delicate parts being properly protected and hoses being loosely coiled to allow for adequate penetration of steam. Prevacuum steam sterilisation is the method of choice for sterilising powered surgical instruments.

STERILISATION

Annabel Herron and Linda Shields

In the health world, the concept of sterilisation is not a new one. In 1864, Louis Pasteur first deduced that the removal of germs stopped putrefaction and Joseph Lister in the late 1800s realised that if this was applied to surgery then rates of infection dropped.[16] Sterilisation is a process by which all forms of microbial life are rendered unable to reproduce; a process used to ensure something is free of all live microorganisms.[17] In early times, methods tried included fire, boiling and immersion in chemicals such as lysol. Over time, and with the development of technology, highly advanced disposable concepts have evolved and these have been particularly useful in the OR. Sterilisation is an important part of the OR process and it is essential that sterilisation processes run efficiently. In many large hospitals, the cleaning, disinfection and sterilisation of equipment are undertaken by the Central Sterilisation and Supply Department (CSSD). Smaller hospitals either use the facilities of larger, nearby hospitals or have developed their own methods of sterilisation according to set standards. The CSSD is responsible for the cleaning, sterilisation and processing of OR instruments and equipment.

METHODS OF STERILISATION OR DISINFECTION

There are several agents used by healthcare facilities to eliminate viable organisms from items (sterilisation). The three methods used for sterilisation in most healthcare facilities are steam under pressure (steam sterilisation), dry heat and low-temperature chemical sterilisation such as ethylene oxide, peracetic acid and plasma sterilisers.

Cleaning instruments before sterilisation

Before sterilisation of instruments can occur, the instruments must be cleaned thoroughly. Standard precautions and the use of personal-protective attire must be used when cleaning instruments. These standards should be followed at all stages to prevent exposure of the handler to blood and body substances.[17] All blood and body substances from all persons are treated as potential sources of infection independent of diagnosis or perceived risk. It is of vital importance that appropriate personal protective gear is worn at all times when handling and cleaning equipment. Heavy-duty (reusable utility) gloves are worn to reduce the risk of hand injuries, specially designed fluid repellent masks, eye protection, faceshields and fluid-resistant aprons or gowns are all available. To ease cleaning, instruments can be placed in water or disinfectant/detergent as soon as possible after use so that debris does not dry onto the instrument.[18]

Routines have been devised to ensure manual cleaning of instruments is thorough. This involves flushing the item in running water between 15 and 30°C to remove visible blood and body substances, then in a sink filled with water and detergent at approximately 45°C. The instruments must be dismantled or opened so that all surfaces are exposed, and lumens and valves are scrubbed using non-lint cloths or non-abrasive scouring pads. Stubborn stains are soaked in a specific stain-removing solution.

Some healthcare facilities have mechanical cleaners for instruments, e.g. a batch-type washer or surgical equipment rack conveyor washer (tunnel washer). Batch-type washers have closed cabinets linked to the water supply and drainage system similar to a household dishwasher, and work in similar cycles to clean the instruments. Tunnel washers operate on a continuous process by means of a conveyor that transports them from stage to stage at a fixed speed in the washer.

The efficiency of cleaning is enhanced with covered ultrasonic cleaners used in particular for sharp instruments so that the risk of personal injury while cleaning such instruments is reduced. The ultrasonic cleaner uses high-frequency, high-energy sound waves that dislodge matter from the instrument, which then drops to the bottom of the cage. Lubrication with a water-soluble solution following ultrasonic cleaning protects them from corrosion.[19] There is some evidence that recontamination occurs after cleaning.[20] **In every case, for all cleaning, it is imperative that manufacturers' instructions for the instruments being cleaned, for the machine or process used for cleaning and for the chemicals used must be closely followed.**[1,21]

Packaging and wrapping

Before sterilisation, items must be dry and packed and wrapped effectively to provide a barrier to prevent contamination, to maintain sterility and to permit aseptic removal of the contents.[17] Packing materials should afford removal of air from the package, permit penetration (and removal) of the sterilising agent and allow water to evaporate.[19] As with all steps of the process, packaging also requires monitoring including the following:

- Integrity of the outer wrap and seals.
- Correct labelling.
- Ease of opening.
- Application of correct techniques for the packaging itself.
- Correct inclusion and layout of contents.
- Cleanliness of the contents.
- Instruments aligned and functioning properly.
- Ability to see if the internal indicator has changed colour when used.

There are many different packaging and wrapping materials available specific to the types of sterilisation processes. They include materials such as textile linen wraps, woven polyester, and paper bags and wraps. Flexible packaging systems are available that are made of materials which can be cellulose-based, porous non-cellulose-based and non-porous non-cellulose-based.[17,21] Rigid, reusable sterilisation container systems include those made of perforated metal, non-perforated metal and perforated plastic.[19]

Before use of any sterilising process, the user should determine if the packs are appropriate for the specific style of sterilisation process. The sealing of packages is of utmost importance in the sterilisation process. Sealing maintains integrity of the pack and inhibits contamination. Heat sealers are used to join the edges and folds, or sterilising indicator tape can be applied. Methods such as staples, pins, incorrect tape or anything that either punctures or does not adhere effectively should not be used.[17] Heat sealing, used on sterilising bags and laminated pouches, compresses the edges of the packet and seals the pack. Sterilising indicator tape can be used to seal packages and, at the same time, indicates the effectiveness of the process by changing colour. There are particular tapes for various uses and the correct one should always be used. Any tape used must be pressure-sensitive, non-toxic, adhere to clean surfaces and be compatible with the chosen wrapping system. It is important that the tape change colour and that the change is distinctly different from the unprocessed tape after exposure to the sterilising agent. Heat-sensitive chemical indicators on their own do not guarantee adequacy of sterilisation, but they act as indicators of those packs that have been processed.[17]

Chemical and biological indicators

It is important to determine if a sterilising process has been effective. Often this is done by placing a chemical indicator placed inside and in the centre of a load of unwrapped instruments or in each instrument pack.[17,21] If the indicator suggests that the process has been inadequate, the contents of the package should not be used. Some internal chemical indicators indicate time and temperature exposure within the package. They should be placed in the area in the package considered least penetrable by the sterilising agent.

STERILISATION METHODS

Steam sterilisation is the most widely used method in healthcare facilities. Heat and moisture maintained at a preset temperature, pressure and time coagulates cell protein and kills the microorganisms present.

Steam under pressure

Steam sterilisation is the most effective and cost-efficient method of sterilisation.[17] Preferably, all heat-stable instruments should be sterilised routinely between uses by steam sterilisation. Steam sterilisation is not toxic, unlike some other methods, but before sterilising any item by steam, it should be ascertained that the item is suitable to go through the extreme heat of the process. Again, specific manufacturer's instructions for both the piece of equipment and the steriliser must be checked. The operator's manual for the steriliser should be available at all times .

Downward displacement: jacket steam sterilisers

Because air is heavier than steam, this type of steriliser acts by allowing pressurised steam in the top of the chamber from the outer jacket, the steam pressure pushes the air to the bottom of the chamber and it releases through a temperature-sensitive valve. Steam builds up in the chamber and the temperature rises until the required temperature is reached and the valve closes. Items must be loaded so that the steam can flow freely around them. If the load is too dense or improperly positioned, pockets of air can be trapped that act as an insulator and the adjacent items will not be effectively sterilised. The cycle will take approximately 30 minutes. The steriliser operates at sterilising temperatures ranging from 121 to 134°C, and the drying cycle time determined by the size and density of the packs.[17]

Downward displacement: emergency 'Flash' steriliser

There is some controversy about the use of so-called 'flash' sterilisation methods and it is widely accepted that this method should be used only for dropped instruments or emergencies. The use of a flash steriliser when time restrictions mean that sterilised packs are not available or there are insufficient instruments for a full list is not appropriate although this is a far too common practice.

Flash sterilisation is suitable for unwrapped, non-porous items only as it has no drying mechanism.[17,21] Flash packs are available for use in a flash steriliser. Instruments can be safely transported from the steriliser to the OR in the flash pack.

Flash sterilising should never be used for blind-ended cannulated instruments and prosthetic implantable devices. All equipment subjected to flash sterilisation must be adequately cleaned, and the process monitored regularly to ensure its efficacy.[17,21] Flash sterilisation has caused injury[22] and care must be taken to ensure the instruments from the steriliser are cool. The steriliser door must **not** be 'cracked', that is the door opened slightly to speed up the cooling process, as it can result in contamination of the load.

Portable steam sterilisers (benchtop sterilisers)

Benchtop sterilisers are appropriate for small healthcare facilities such as doctor, surgeries and private clinics. Small quantities of wrapped and unwrapped small items can be effectively sterilised. During a cycle, water is boiled in the chamber space, steam is generated which expels the chamber air and the chamber heats to the required temperature.[17]

Prevacuum sterilisers

Air is withdrawn by vacuum from the sterilising chamber and steam injected, giving greater steam penetration in a short time.[17] After the required time, steam is removed through a filter and the temperature and pressure in the chamber reduced. This cycle takes approximately 5 minutes with temperatures between 134 and 136°C.

Low-temperature sterilisers and liquid sterilants

Some equipment is not suitable for sterilisation with any process that is heat dependent. These include instruments such as telescopes, fibreoptic light leads, and flexible endoscopes, bronchoscopes and colonoscopes. The manufacturer's directions about concentration and exposure time should be followed closely, and all details of the liquid chemical agent (sterilant/disinfectant) will be shown on the label.[17] Material Safety Data Sheets (MSDS) must be available for all chemicals used.

Types of chemical sterilisation and disinfection

Ethylene oxide gas kills microorganisms by destroying the normal metabolism of protein and reproductive processes in cells.[17] It is used for heat- and moisture-sensitive items such as plastics, fibreoptics and materials that corrode.[23] Ethylene oxide permeates porous material and leaves no film. Such sterilisation can be expensive as the process can be complicated and lengthy. All gas residue must be allowed to evaporate as a potentially carcinogenic toxic gas is released during and after the process. Ethylene oxide gas is highly flammable. All staff using the gas must have yearly health checks, and safety procedures must be known and implemented.[1,19]

Temperature plasma sterilisers

Low-temperature plasma sterilisation provides a safer alternative to ethylene oxide gas sterilisation. It can also be used on heat- and pressure-sensitive items. While the physics of the process is beyond the scope of this book, in summary hydrogen peroxide gas is converted to a plasma by exposure to microwave energy in a vacuum, while within the plasma, hydrogen peroxide is broken into particles that interact with cell membranes, thereby killing microorganisms.[17] By-products from the process are water and oxygen. On completion of the cycle, the sterilising chamber is returned to atmospheric pressure by the introduction of filtered air. It can be used with items with narrow lumens (a special adapter is needed), and wrapping material must be non-woven polypropylene. Paper-wrapping materials cannot be used with this process and all instruments and equipment must be completely dry or damage can occur during the sterilising process. The cycle takes about 75 minutes and aeration of packages is required.

Plasma sterilisation is a cheap alternative to ethylene oxide and formaldehyde,[24] and is just as effective in killing microorganisms.[25] However, it has been associated with toxic endothelial cell destruction syndrome in ophthalmic patients, where it causes degradation of metals used in the manufacture of the operating instruments which in turn can cause damage to the eye tissues.[26]

Glutaraldehyde

Glutaraldehyde is dealt with in depth in Chapter 5.

Peracetic acid-sterilising equipment

The Steris™ System uses peracetic acid (vinegar) to kill bacteria at 50°C.[17] The system has a sealed chamber in which peracetic acid is diluted to a 0.2% solution and heated to between 50 and 55°C. The cycle runs for 12 minutes and automatically drains off all the fluid once the solution has been neutralised by the automatic injection of a buffering agent into the chamber.[17] Items are then rinsed in sterile water. Steris™ sterilises immersible surgical and diagnostic items. As with all sterilising techniques, it is effective only if cleaning has been adequate before immersion. Instruments with a lumen and other possible contamination traps must be cleaned with bacteriostatic or protein neutraliser product. Steris™ is of particular use in the sterilisation of scopes, and research has indicated that while it is more expensive than other methods, it is less toxic than glutaraldehyde and it is usually more effective.[27-30]

MONITORING STERILITY
Mechanical indicators

All sterilising machines have in-built gauges, thermometers, timers, recorders, function monitors and alarm systems. However, daily test runs using prescribed formulae and processes are necessary to ensure adequate sterilising and efficient working of

Infection control

the system. Guidelines in manuals relating to the maintenance and running of each system should be adhered to, as must policies and procedures laid down in each OR, CSSD and health facility.

Chemical indicators are used to determine that the correct parameters of time and temperature have been reached during the sterilisation process. Indicators include colour tapes, and dyes impregnated into materials. It is important for OR staff to be aware of the indicators used in their unit and how to interpret their readings.[19]

Biological indicators

'A biological indicator is a population of calibrated bacterial spores on, or in, a carrier which is packaged in such a manner that the integrity of the inoculated carrier is maintained'[17] (p. 11). Biological indicators can be strips placed in the load or small plastic pellets containing living spores. After going through the sterilising process, they are incubated to determine the level of resistant microorganism growth.[1,17] If any organisms have survived the sterilising process, this indicates a fault in the steriliser. All items processed in that load must be recalled and another test run with biological indicators must be carried out. Records of the performance of each steriliser in a facility should be kept as well as the details of each cycle.[1]

EMERGING PROBLEMS: CREUTZFELDT–JAKOB DISEASE

In the final years of the last century, the emergence of AIDS brought about a rethinking of sterilising and infection control practices, and the implementation of 'universal' and now 'standard' precautions. However, in the past few years, a new disease has emerged which is producing anxiety in any health field in which any sort of contamination can occur. Creutzfeldt–Jakob disease (CJD) has been recognised since the 1920s,[30] but it is only recently that its mode of transmission and relationship to the animal diseases bovine spongiform encephalitis (BSE, or 'mad cow disease') and scrapie (an illness in sheep) has been discovered. While transmission is not fully understood, it is known that a section of a protein called a 'prion' is responsible for carrying the disease.[31] As this is not a single, living organism, as is a bacterium or a

virus, rather, a 'bit' of broken-down matter, sterilising by known, conventional methods may not render the material harmless. Research continues into the best way of preventing nosocomial spread of this disease, and the most reliable method would be to use only disposable instruments in surgery. This, of course, is not practical and would be immensely costly, so guidelines are being drawn up and evaluated to find the best way to prevent contamination. Because of the mode of transmission, normal sterilisation methods are not sufficient.[32,33]

Various organisations around the world such as the National Health and Medical Research Council of Australia[34] and the Centers for Disease Control and Prevention[35] and numerous infection control organisations are continuously monitoring and developing infection control guidelines for this most insidious disease. However, the best way to prevent contamination in the OR is preparedness. By knowing about the condition, its mode of spread and by having guidelines already prepared and the staff educated to use the guidelines, then patients in your OR will be less at risk.[31]

References

1. *Standards and Recommended Practices*. Denver: Association of Operating Room Nurses, 1993.
2. Meeker RH, Rothrock, JC. *Alexander's Care of the Patient in Surgery*, 11th edn. St Louis: Mosby, 1995.
3. Parker L. From pestilence to asepsis. *Nurs Times* 1990; 49: 63–67.
4. Rhodes P. *An Outline of the History of Medicine*. London: Butterworths, 1985.
5. Goldsmith I, Lip GY, Khan F, Hutton R, Patel RL. Contamination of the surgeon's bare and gloved fingertips in cardiac operations. *Int J Clin Pract* 1998; 52: 529–532.
6. Jeray KJ, Banks DM, Phieffer LS, Middlebrooks ES, Frankenburg KP, Hudson, MC, Kellam, JF, Bosse MJ. Evaluation of standard surgical preparation performed on superficial dermal abrasions. *J Orthop Trauma* 2000; 14: 206–211.
7. Poon C, Morgan DJ, Pond F, Kane J, Tulloh BR. Studies of the surgical scrub. *Aust N Z J Surg* 1998; 68: 65–67.
8. Loeb MB, Wilcox L, Smaill F, Walter S, Duff Z. A randomized trial of surgical scrubbing with a brush compared to antiseptic soap alone. *Am J Infect Control* 1997; 25: 11–15.
9. Hobson DW, Woller W, Anderson L, Guthery E. Development and evaluation of a new alcohol-based surgical hand scrub formulation with persistent antimicrobial characteristics and brushless application. *Am J Infect Control* 1998; 26: 507–512.

10. Anttonen H, Puhakka K, Niskanen J, Ryhanen P. Cutaneous heat loss in children during anaesthesia. *Br J Anaesth* 1995; 74: 306–310.

11. Belkin NL, Koch FT. OR barrier materials – necessity or extravagance? *AORN J* 1998; 67: 443–445.

12. Blacklock BJ. Over-draping: a practice question. *Can Oper Room Nurs J* 1996; 14: 9–11.

13. Bolton DT. Ophthalmic draping and carbon dioxide retention [Letter] *Anaesthesia* 1999; 54: 1230–1231.

14. Reid JS, Wilson SC. Draping of the pelvis and proximal femur: an improved method for applying self-adherent plastic drapes. *Am J Orthop* 1997; 26: 229, 232–233.

15. Phippen ML, Wells MP. *Patient Care During Operative and Invasive Procedures.* Philadelphia: WB Saunders, 2000.

16. Poynter FNL, Keele KD, Goodier J. *A Short History of Medicine.* London: Scientific Book Club, 1961.

17. Standards Australia. *Australian Standard AS 4187 (1998) Code of Practice for Cleaning, Disinfecting and Sterilising Reusable Medical and Surgical Instruments and Equipment Maintenance of Associated Environments in Health Care Facilities.* Homebush: Standards Australia, 1998.

18. Merritt K, Hitchins VM, Brown SA. Safety and cleaning of medical materials and devices. *J Biomed Mater Res* 2000; 53: 131–136.

19. Rhyne L, Ulmer BC, Revell L. Monitoring and controlling the environment. In: Phippen ML, Wells MP. *Patient Care during Operative and Invasive Procedures.* Philadelphia: WB Saunders, 2000.

20. Chu NS, Chan-Myers H, Ghazanfari N, Antonoplos P. Levels of naturally occurring microorganisms on surgical instruments after clinical use and after washing. *Am J Infect Control* 1999; 27: 315–319.

21. Association of Operating Room Nurses. Recommended practices for the care and cleaning of surgical instruments and powered equipment. *AORN J* 1997; 65: 124–128.

22. Rutala WA, Weber DJ, Chappell KJ. Patient injury from flash-sterilized instruments [Letter]. *Infect Control Hosp Epidemiol* 1999; 20: 458.

23. *Infection Control in the Health Care Setting: Guidelines for the Prevention of Transmission of Infectious Diseases.* Canberra: National Health and Medical Research Council of Australia, 1996.

24. Adler S, Scherrer M, Daschner FD. Costs of low-temperature plasma sterilization compared with other sterilization methods. *J Hosp Infect* 1998; 40: 125–134.

25. Kyi MS, Holton J, Ridgway GL. Assessment of the efficacy of a low temperature hydrogen peroxide gas plasma sterilization system. *J Hosp Infect* 1995; 31: 275–284.

26. Duffy RE, Brown SE, Caldwell KL, Lubniewski A, Anderson N, Edelhauser H, Holley G, Tess A, Divan H, Helmy M, Arduino M, Jarvis WR. An epidemic of corneal destruction caused by plasma gas sterilization. *Arch Ophthalmol* 2000; 118: 1167–1176.

27. Tandon RK, Ahuja V. Non-United States guidelines for endoscope reprocessing. *Gastrointest Endosc Clin N Am* 2000; 10: 295–318.

28. Society of Gastroenterology Nurses and Associates. Guideline for the use of high-level disinfectants and sterilants for reprocessing of flexible gastrointestinal endoscopes. *Gastroenterol Nurs* 1999; 22: 127–134.

29. Cronmiller JR, Nelson DK, Jackson DK, Kim CH. Efficacy of conventional endoscopic disinfection and sterilization methods against *Helicobacter pylori* contamination. *Helicobacter* 1999; 4: 198–203.

30. Vesley D, Melson J, Stanley P. Microbial bioburden in endoscope reprocessing and an in-use evaluation of the high-level disinfection capabilities of Cidex PA *Gastroenterol Nurs* 1999; 22: 63–68.

31. Hansel PA. Mad cow disease: the OR connection. *AORN J* 1999; 70: 224–238.

32. Mocsny N. The spongiform encephalopathies: prion diseases. *J Neurosci Nurs* 1998; 30: 302–306.

33. Dormont D. How to limit the spread of Creutzfeldt–Jakob disease. *Infect Control Hosp Epidemiol* 1996; 17: 521–528.

34. National Health and Medical Research Council. *Creutzfeldt–Jakob disease and other human transmissible spongiform encephalopathies*, 2001. Available from URL: http://www.health.gov.au/nhmrc/publicat/pdf/ic5.pdf

35. Centers for Disease Control and Infection Healthcare Infection Control Practices Advisory Committee. *Draft guideline for environmental infection control in healthcare facilities*, 2001. Available from URL: http://www.cdc.gov/ncidod/hip/enviro/env_guide_draft.pdf

4 | Instruments

Maria Anderson

USE OF SURGICAL INSTRUMENTS

Anthropological evidence from the dawn of history reveals the use of cranial trepanning. The skull roof was opened with sharpened flint blades, with no real knowledge of anatomy and no aseptic technique. Human skulls clearly showed healing of the surrounding bony tissue and the person survived long after the surgical intervention.[1]

With the Iron and Bronze Ages came the ability to forge surgical tools such as scalpels, hooks, dilators and probes, to name a few. These were used to remove limbs, probe abscesses and to 'let blood'. Both the Egyptian and Roman civilisations used surgical instruments.[2] All these procedures were conducted without anaesthetics and aseptic techniques, which were not invented until the late 19th century.[3] In the 21st century, advanced surgical instruments are part of the overall picture of modern medicine. While the following is a basic overview of the instruments that might be found in a basic surgical tray, there is a huge variety of instruments used in many varied surgical specialities.

It is imperative that the operating room (OR) nurse is aware of the care and handling of surgical instruments as their cost is often very high and department budgets will not allow for excessive repair or replacement of damaged instruments. The life of an instrument can be reduced drastically when it is used incorrectly, therefore it is important for the OR nurse to know the names of the instruments and their appropriate use. During the instrument tray check, it is important to examine the instruments for any damage and wear. Defective instruments should be removed from the tray as they may inhibit progress of the surgery and cause unnecessary damage to the patient.

The following instruments are commonly used in all ORs.

Sponge-holding forceps

Description: long-handled forceps with broad ends.
  Uses:

- To hold the preparation swabs.
- To hold a swab for touching bleeding points.
- As a retractor, with a small swab wrapped around the tip. It is used to keep tissues away from the working area. It is commonly called 'swab on a stick'.

Inspect: for cleanliness, hinges and joints work smoothly, the ratchet mechanism allows the jaws to close smoothly and maintain their closed position.

Towel clips

Description: to hold drapes in place, though with modern disposable adhesive drapes they are rapidly becoming an instrument of the past. Towel clips have

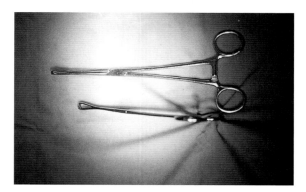

Fig. 4.1 Sponge-holding forceps

5 | Safety measures

Helen Werder and Andrea Thompson

All staff working within the perioperative area must adhere to their respective statutory requirements and hospital policy for their safety programmes. Each perioperative area should have active personnel on committees such as Occupational Health & Safety, Quality Improvement and Infection Control. Participation in such groups promotes standards within the unit that employ critical thinking about current and topical issues relating to quality outcomes and safety for patients and staff. All personnel working in perioperative areas should be aware of the hazards peculiar to operating room (OR) activities and working conditions.[1]

Safety measures should be employed in the areas of fire and electrical safety, electrosurgery, radiation monitoring, laser usage, protection from needlestick injuries and substance splashes, and the handling and storage of volatile liquids/hazardous substances.

FIRE AND ELECTRICAL SAFETY

Helen Werder

Electrical and fire regulations should be formulated for each operating suite by that hospital's administration and the management of the operating suite. The perioperative management team should then delegate the responsibility and authority to ensure that the regulations are maintained by all OR staff members.[1] These regulations should include the following.

- Fire evacuation plan that has been endorsed by the Fire and Security Department of that hospital.
- Regular fire evacuation practice programme that includes all members of the operative team.
- Nominated fire warden for the perioperative area for each shift.

- Identification of the fire exits and an in-service programme for the staff in the use of fire extinguishers within the perioperative area.
- Non-smoking policy and a ban on the use of any open flame device within the area.
- All new equipment should be inspected and evaluated to ensure optimum safety and performance.
- Routine maintenance and electrical inspection programmes should be maintained within the area.
- Biomechanical technicians should have the authority to determine whether any electrical equipment, lights and electrosurgical units are safe for use in a given situation.
- Personnel should be given instruction about the use and care of all electrical equipment and should demonstrate their competence in return.
- All electrical equipment should have an adeq length of electrical cord attached to reach the outlet without strain and without the use of extension cords.
- Personnel should inspect the plug, cord and con tions of all electrical equipment before usage.
- When plugging electrical equipment int removing from the socket, the plug and not the cord should be used.
- Cords should be coiled loosely when not in u avoid breaking the internal wiring.
- Beds and other equipment should not be pu over electrical cords on the floor.
- Cords which of necessity are on the floor w staff are walking should be taped down to avoid staff tripping over them.
- All personnel should be familiar with procedures for prompt removal from use and repair processing for damaged or faulty equipment.

Hazardous situations in ORs are caused by the combination of faulty electrical equipment and combustible materials found in the area. Most anaesthetic gases used now are non-combustible and conductive flooring and footwear is no longer required. If a volatile agent is still in use and conductive flooring is still employed, then annual testing and reporting on the safety of this flooring is still required.

Banks of electrical outlets are fitted with a core balance unit that will close down power to that bank of outlets if a faulty piece of electrical equipment is plugged in. If this occurs, the last piece of equipment plugged in or the faulty piece of equipment must be identified and removed for testing and repair. If the core balance unit cannot be reset, then the theatre must be closed after that patient's surgery is completed and electrical maintenance carried out on that unit.

VOLATILE LIQUIDS/HAZARDOUS SUBSTANCES

All flammable and volatile liquids and hazardous substances must be properly stored, managed and controlled within the workplace in accordance with current workplace health and safety legislation and the relevant dangerous goods code. Flammable liquids should be stored in a flammable liquids' cupboard, which should not be in a public place or in a public thoroughfare.

In a location adjacent to the cupboard or in an area readily accessible to all staff should be stored a manifest and the Material Safety Data Sheets (MSDSs) for chemicals and solutions kept in the perioperative area. Each manufacturer of the chemical or solution is required to provide safety information relevant to that solution. Staff should be familiar with the contents of the information sheets. Annual audits should be conducted to ensure the manifest is current, the MSDSs are held for all solutions, and that staff are current in their training requirements and that personal protective equipment (PPE) is provided for the handling of the hazardous substances.

Skin-preparation solutions should be carefully applied to avoid pooling of the solutions, which may cause a chemical burn and prevent drying of the solution on the skin. Accumulated vapours from these solutions can be ignited by a spark from an active electrode from the electrosurgical unit or a charge of static electricity. When an electrosurgical unit is used, the preparation solution should be non-flammable.

GLUTARALDEHYDE

Aldehydes remain at present the most effective and cost-effective group of chemicals for high-level disinfection of semicritical items.[2] Semicritical items include items that come into contact with intact skin or mucous membranes and should be free of microorganisms except for spores. Semicritical items include fibreoptic scopes and associated equipment that will be present at the operative field, e.g. anaesthetic equipment, bronchoscopes, gastrointestinal endoscopes and kermometers. It follows that arthroscopes, hysteroscopes, laparoscopes and their accessories, cystoscopes and all other instruments entering normally sterile locations in the body must have been processed by a recognised sterilisation method.[2] Aldehydes are the most common alternative for high-level disinfection of equipment that cannot be sterilised by high-pressure, high-temperature steam sterilisation but can be exposed to moisture and unable for whatever constraints, be it time or convenience, to go through the process of ethylene oxide.

The perioperative nurse should be aware of the health risks when using aldehydes to maintain safe practice. Aldehydes may have two main effects, irritation and allergy, and several other symptoms on humans. The symptoms of irritation may be as given in table 5.1.

The symptoms of allergy may be those outlined in table 5.2.

Other symptoms may be those outlined in table 5.3.

The occupational exposure standard for glutaraldehyde varies between 0.1 and 0.2 parts per million (ppm).[3–5] This is a peak concentration that should not be exceeded. It should be noted that an increase in temperature of glutaraldehyde increases its disinfection properties and increases the fumes and vapour emitted.

Worksafe Australia Hazard Alert No. 1 (October 1991) stated:

Table 5.1
Symptoms of irritation caused by glutaraldehyde

- Contact dermatitis
- Sore, gritty, burning eyes and/or conjunctivitis
- Nasal, throat irritations, rhinitis, epistaxis
- Headaches
- Nausea
- Chest tightness

Table 5.2
Symptoms of allergy caused by glutaraldehyde

- Allergic dermatitis to exposed areas including the face and arms
- Allergic rhinitis and asthma, and in cases of prolonged exposure
- Damage to the vocal cords and loss of sensation in the mouth, throat and oesophagus have occurred

Table 5.3
Other adverse symptoms caused by glutaraldehyde

- Chronic fatigue
- Loss of appetite
- Headache and nausea

Glutaraldehyde liquids, aerosols and vapour can act as an irritant and sensitiser to the skin and the airways of the respiratory tract:

- *appropriate ventilation*
- *work practices*
- *personal protective equipment (PPE)*

are required to prevent skin contact and inhalation.[6]

Appropriate ventilation

All areas where glutaraldehyde is used should be properly ventilated. This may be by means of controlled airflow that exhausts to atmosphere or by purpose designed recirculating fume cabinets with activated charcoal chemical vapour-absorbent filters. If recirculating fume cabinets are being used, their ability to maintain adequately low levels of vapour glutaraldehyde in the breathing zone of operator(s) needs to be tested before installation. Where ventilation cannot control the operator's exposure to glutaraldehyde from inhalation, additional PPE such as a respirator may be necessary.

Whichever ventilation method is used, an air-sampling assessment by the appropriate authorities of the measure of the concentration of glutaraldehyde vapour in the operator's normal breathing zone is necessary when an installation is first completed. This should be a once-only process, but repeated testing is needed when there is a variation in the equipment, layout or ventilation system surrounding a situation of use of glutaraldehyde.

Monitoring of the reliable operation of ventilation systems, knowledge of the effectiveness of recirculating fume cabinets and/or observance of the recommended regimen for replacement of activated charcoal filters (where used) assures the continuing minimisation of hazard to workers due to glutaraldehyde vapour in the breathing space.[2]

Work practices

Containers containing glutaraldehyde should be covered at all times when instruments or equipment are not being placed into or retrieved from them. This helps prevent evaporation into the atmosphere, which alters the composition of the solution, exposes personnel to fumes and contaminates the solution with airborne particles.[7]

Glutaraldehyde should be used according to the manufacturer's instructions. Written instruction sheets and the chemical/hazard sheet need to be readily available for staff perusal at the site of storage and activation.

Instruments and equipment to be disinfected should be thoroughly cleaned with an enzymatic cleaner detergent to remove organic matter and dried before immersion in glutaraldehyde. Biological matter remaining on instrumentation prevents effective disinfection of the affected surface by the solution. Wet items placed in the glutaraldehyde solution will dilute the chemical strength thus reducing its effectiveness. Items with lumens, channels and crevices must be irrigated with the solution. Items should be disinfected before each use and before storage.

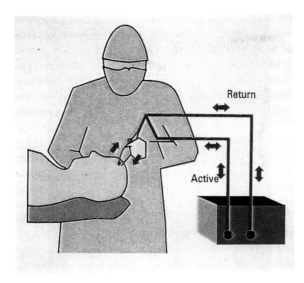

Fig. 5.3 Bipolar circuit

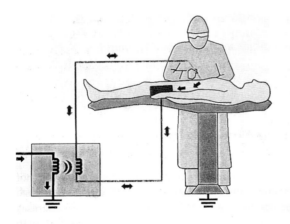

Fig. 5.4 Isolated electrosurgical systems

Safety precautions

Before using an electrosurgical unit in the operating theatre, the theatre personnel should be competent in utilising the use of this equipment to provide safety to the patient and theatre personnel.

These precautions consist of the following.

- Ensuring the staff receive sufficient education and assessment in the use of electrosurgical equipment.

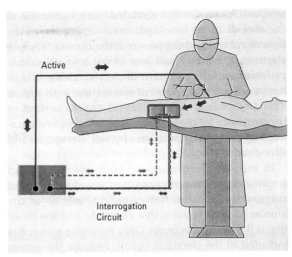

Fig. 5.5 REM circuit

- Ensuring the electrosurgical unit is scheduled for regular maintenance.
- Checking that cables and electrodes have regular insulation checks.
- Ensuring that the skin integrity of the patient is checked before and after use of the electrosurgical unit, especially under the dispersive electrode.[1]
- Ensuring the active electrode (diathermy pencil or forceps) is placed in a clean, dry, non-conductive safety holster in a highly visible area when not in use during the procedure.[10]
- Ensuring that single-use active and return electrodes are not reused.
- Placing the return electrode on an area free from hair, skin lesions, blemishes or scars.
- Placing the return electrode as close to the operative site as is practical.
- Applying the return electrode over a vascular, muscular area to encourage heat dissipation under the return electrode.
- Ensuring the entire area of the return electrode is in direct and complete contact with the patient. If the patient is moved during surgery, it is necessary to recheck the return electrode site.
- Ensuring the return electrode remains dry during surgery and precautions should be taken to prevent pooling of flammable liquids in any cavity, under the body or on the return electrode itself.

- Ensuring the patient does not come into contact with any grounded object.
- Checking that the return electrode is entirely covered with gel before application.
- In conjunction with the surgeon and the manufacturer's recommendations, the settings for use of the electrosurgical unit should be as low as possible.
- Checking all possible causes for faults if the return electrode-monitoring system deactivates the electrosurgical unit intraoperatively.
- Using a smoke-evacuation system to remove the electrosurgical plume from the operating theatre.

RADIATION SAFETY

Exposure to ionising radiation can cause damage to living tissues and may have longer-term cumulative effects. Personnel working in the perioperative area must protect their patients and themselves from exposure to this type of radiation. The radiology department and the perioperative nurse share this responsibility.

Recommended practices to minimise the amount of radiation exposure consist of the following.

- Identifying at risk patients, e.g. pregnant women, and covering the foetus and reproductive organs with a lead gown if possible during radiology screening.
- Covering perioperative personnel with PPE, which would include lead aprons, thyroid protectors, eyewear and gloves during exposure to X-rays.
- Encouraging all personnel who can leave the room during screening to do so as increasing distance from the X-ray source decreases exposure dosage.
- Providing leaded screens for scrubbed personnel who cannot leave the operating theatre environment.
- Ensuring personnel covered in protective equipment do not position themselves so that unprotected parts of their anatomy face the X-ray unit.
- Using positioning equipment to maintain the patient's position during the screening period.

Perioperative personnel who have frequent exposure to radiation should wear radiation-monitoring devices, which should be worn on the same part of the body each use and be read by a qualified radiation-monitoring service.

Leaded protective devices should be handled carefully and hung correctly to prevent damage to the leaded material. The aprons should be screened periodically to detect damage not seen by visual inspection. Personnel who treat patients who have received diagnostic or therapeutic radionuclides should protect themselves:

- by limiting the amount of time spent in close proximity to the patient;[10] and
- by handling body fluids and tissue from the patients according to radiation safety procedures.

Personnel who handle therapeutic radiation sources should beep the radioactive material in its transport container until insertion into the patient. The material should be handled carefully with forceps.

Policies and procedures should be established in the perioperative area to provide guidelines for training personnel in radiation-protective procedures, for maintenance of protective equipment and for monitoring compliance with safety standards.

PATHOLOGY SPECIMEN HANDLING

Specimens collected during operations are an extremely important responsibility for the operating theatre staff as correct diagnosis and treatment of the patient results from the outcomes obtained. Specimens may be fresh for frozen section, fresh specimens where no preservative is added or preserved in an additive such as formalin (formaldehyde).

It is the responsibility of the operating theatre staff to label the specimen correctly with the date and time of collection, the patient's identification, the name of the surgeon, the patient's ward, the specimen description and to accompany it with the appropriate pathology request form. The care of the specimen will be according to the protocol established by the laboratory of each hospital. Specimens for frozen section must be transported immediately to the laboratory as the operative team may determine the extent of surgery from the reports. Fresh specimens must be transported as soon as possible. Specimens in a preservative may be transported at routine collection rounds.

As all specimens are considered a potential source of infection, the theatre staff must handle them correctly. Staff should wear correct protective equipment such as gloves, masks and protective eyewear when handling specimens and when adding formalin to a specimen. All specimen containers must be kept clean on the outside and placed either in biohazard bags or in an impervious plastic bag to prevent contamination to the personnel transporting them. All specimens must be documented in the patient's operative records and in the pathology specimen book, which provides a record of specimens taken in the operating theatres and of specimens sent to the Pathology Department. This record should include the date and type of specimen, the patient's name, the surgeon's name, and the signature of the staff member recording the specimen. All collection or transporting personnel must sign for receipt of the specimen.

EXPOSURE TO SIGNIFICANT BODY FLUIDS AND SHARPS INJURIES

Personnel working within the perioperative area are at significant risk of being exposed to body fluids and of receiving injuries from sharp instruments and needles. By identifying work practices that put personnel at risk and providing guidelines to minimise this risk, the staff and patients can significantly reduce this risk.

PERSONAL RISK PROTECTION

The application of the principles of universal precautions including the use of protective barriers, hand washing, and care in the use and disposal of needles and other sharp instruments should be used for all invasive procedures.[10] Application of these principles should minimise the risk of transmission of human immunodeficiency virus (HIV), hepatitis viruses and other blood-borne pathogens between patients and healthcare personnel.

Included in these precautions to reduce the risk to healthcare personnel should be the following.

- Wearing of PPE such as goggles or glasses with side shields, face shields, masks, gowns and gloves. Double gloving is now recommended in most practice settings. The risk of exposure will dictate the type and characteristics of PPE used.
- Use of containers for scalpels and needle holders with sutures when passing these between the scrub nurse and the surgeon.
- Careful handling when removing and disposing of all sharps at the end of the surgical procedure.
- Disposal of sharp items such as scalpel blades and sutures into a sterile sharps container intraoperatively and then into a larger sharps biohazard container postoperatively.
- Discouraging of the recapping of needles, but when unavoidable, it should be carried out with the aid of mechanical devices.
- Refraining of personnel who have open lesions from working in a situation or area that places them at risk of exposure to contamination.
- Wearing of PPE when handling specimens.
- Wearing of PPE when cleaning equipment, instruments or disposing of suction equipment liners.
- Use by the surgeon of blunt or extra blunt needles when closing the abdominal wall fascia.[1]
- Receiving of hepatitis B immunisation before occupational exposure occurs.

ACCIDENTAL EXPOSURE

If healthcare workers sustain accidental exposure to body fluids or a sharps injury, there should be in place in every facility a protocol for the staff member to follow. The exposure should be reported immediately to personnel in a supervisory position and the staff member should cleanse the site thoroughly of any contaminating body fluids. Following the policy and procedures, the staff member should receive prompt intervention, testing, counselling and any other appropriate prophylaxis.[10] The details of the incident should be recorded for possible worker's compensation claims or other litigation.

All staff should receive education about these policies and procedures during orientation to enable them to develop knowledge, skills and a safe attitude to work practice to help reduce exposure to occupational risks. These policies and procedures should be reviewed regularly within the workplace to provide safe guidelines for all personnel.

LASER SAFETY

The introduction of laser technology into the surgical arena has witnessed its application in a wide range of surgical specialities. 'The laser has radically changed surgery by making possible less invasive procedures, thus decreasing inpatient hospitalisation, diminishing postoperative complications, and saving healthcare dollars'[1] (p. 1245). The perioperative nurse has expanded responsibilities with laser application and it is important that there exists within each organisation a set of generic basic guidelines for its use.

'Laser' is an acronym for *light amplification by the stimulated emission of radiation*. There are many different types of lasers, namely ruby crystal, argon, carbon dioxide, ND:Yag, holmium, and diode lasers, and others are being developed. Laser technology has provided a precision tool for cutting, coagulating, vaporising and welding tissue during surgical intervention.[1] Laser describes the generator itself and the process in which light energy is produced.

Light is a form of electromagnetic energy measured in wavelengths extending from the shorter waves in the ultraviolet area to the longer waves in the infrared region along a perpetual line. The visible wavelengths occupy only a small portion of this continuum. 'The radiation of laser technology is nonionizing in that it does not present the hazard of cellular DNA disruption through continual tissue exposure' and is therefore not harmful to pregnant staff[1] (p. 1245). 'A laser beam is created by stimulating photons inside a resonating chamber. As the photons bounce back and forth, they gain energy, which is emitted through the delivery system, producing a laser beam that can be used to cut or coagulate tissue'[11] (p. 353).

Four interactions occur when laser energy is delivered to the target area: reflection, scattering, transmission or absorption. The extent of the reaction of the beam on the target depends on the laser wavelength, power settings, spot size, length of time the beam is in contact with the tissue and the characteristics of the tissue.

- Reflection: occurs when the direction of the beam is changed after it contacts an area. When the angle of the incoming light is equal to the angle of the reflected light, then a specular reflection occurs. This reflection of laser light can be used in difficult-to-access areas by reflecting the laser light off a mirror. Danger can occur if the light is not controlled at all times and the uncontrolled reflected light hits an undesired target.
- Scattering: occurs when the beam spreads over a large area as the tissue causes the beam to disperse. The beam intensity is decreased as the waves scatter in different directions.
- Transmission: occurs when the beam passes through clear fluids or tissue without causing thermal alteration in the fluid or tissue. The argon beam can be transmitted through the fluids and structures of the eye to cause photocoagulation of the retina.
- Absorption: results when the tissue is altered from the impact of the beam. Absorption of the laser beam is affected by the laser wavelength and consistency, colour, and water content of the target tissue. The argon laser light is highly absorbed by pigmented tissues, whereas the carbon dioxide laser is independent of colour-selective absorption.

TYPES OF LASER

Although there are a variety of lasers available, there are three most commonly associated with surgery: carbon dioxide, ND:Yag and argon. Each has benefits and is specific to different types of surgery.

Carbon dioxide laser

The carbon dioxide laser using molecules of carbon dioxide as the lasing medium is the most versatile laser as it can perform both cutting and coagulation of tissues and can be used in both the pulsed and continuous modes of operation. By the variation of the length and frequency of each pulse, different tissue effects can be produced and thermal effects can be more precisely controlled.[11] The carbon dioxide beam can be focused to vaporise a precise amount of tissue or defocused to coagulate tissue. As the carbon dioxide laser wavelength is absorbed by water, and the body is 75–90% water, an extremely precise beam can vaporise a small area while avoiding surrounding tissue.[11] Because the carbon dioxide laser affects only the intended tissue, there is less postoperative pain and faster recovery. This laser can be used in ear, nose and throat (ENT) surgery, gynaecological surgery, plastic surgery, general surgery and neurosurgery.

ND:Yag laser

The ND:Yag laser uses a solid crystal made of *yttrium aluminium garnet* (Yag) covered with *neodymium* (ND) as the active medium. Electrons are excited by a bright, flashing lamp striking the neodymium, which causes a mini-explosion. This laser is used for coagulation and provides a greater penetration depth, but the energy is not highly focused. The laser can be applied using a fibre or contact probe and is suitable for use in endoscopic surgery and ophthalmology.

Argon laser

The argon laser uses gas as its medium but at a different wavelength from the carbon dioxide laser. This argon laser is used in ophthalmology, dermatology, gastroenterology, gynaecology and otology. The beam is absorbed by pigmented tissue whilst passing through clear structures and is commonly used in day surgery settings.

BENEFITS OF LASER

Laser surgery is still an expanding area within the perioperative area but already definite benefits for the patient have become evident. Some of these benefits are the following.

- Production of minimal tissue damage.
- Decrease in the amount of scarring especially in the larynx, which reduces the amount of stenosis.
- Decrease in the amount of postoperative pain.
- Reduction in recovery time and a faster return to daily activities.
- Reduction in the length of surgery and therefore anaesthetic time.
- Increase in the use of local versus general anaesthesia.
- Ability to seal small blood vessels, lymphatics and selected nerve endings.[1]

LASER SAFETY AND CREDENTIALLING

Laser systems can concentrate high amounts of energy within very small areas and therefore have the potential to be hazardous without careful use and speciality training. It is the responsibility of all the perioperative team to receive this training and to ensure its application during laser use. Each country has specific legislative requirements that need to be met by the different members of the health team and it is the responsibility of the hospital to formulate policy and procedures to meet the guidelines for regulation of laser usage. Most of the lasers in use are in surgical procedures and can cause thermal reactions that can lead to fire, skin burns and optical damage by either direct or scattered radiation.[1] Safety precautions must be followed to prevent injury to staff and patients from these laser systems. Nursing staff need to attend special education programmes to understand the energy characteristics of laser light, its clinical application, safety requirements and specific information related to application of the medium within the operative area.

PERIOPERATIVE NURSING CONSIDERATIONS

Perioperative nurses working with laser technology should be aware of the potential hazards to all staff and the patient and ensure a safe environment by performing the following see table 5.4.

- Placing a warning sign appropriate to the type of laser being used on all doors leading into and out of the laser area to alert all personnel that they need to adhere to precautionary measures.
- Covering windows or ports with the appropriate protection for the specific laser wavelength being used.
- Storing the laser key in a safe area but not with the laser machine.
- Keeping the laser in standby mode when not in use.
- Supplying and making sure that all staff are wearing special glasses/goggles applicable to the medium being used, e.g.
  - clear: CO_2 laser;
  - green tint: ND:Yag laser; or
  - orange tint: argon laser.

Table 5.4
AORN recommended practices for laser safety

1. All healthcare workers should be aware of areas of laser use, and controlled access to these areas must be maintained
2. Eyes of patients and healthcare workers should be protected from laser beams
3. Skin and other tissue of patients and healthcare workers should be protected from aberrant and reflected laser beams
4. Patients and healthcare workers should be protected from inhaling the plume associated with laser use
5. Patients and healthcare workers should be protected from fire hazards associated with laser use
6. Patients and healthcare workers should be protected from electrical hazards associated with laser use
7. Laser team should be available within the practice setting
8. Perioperative personnel working in a laser treatment area should be required to obtain safety training and basic orientation to the technology
9. Policies and procedures for laser safety should be developed with regard to the practice setting

---

These glasses/goggles should be inscribed with the correct wavelength protection and optical density for the specific wavelength being used. They should be stored safely so that the surfaces are not scratched as this destroys the effectiveness of the eyewear. Precautions in use include:

- Ensuring the patient's eyes are protected, and that damp sponges are used for protection when using the CO_2 laser to prevent fire ignition. If the patient is awake, then appropriate eyewear and an explanation of the procedure should be given.
- Covering the eyepiece of the endoscope with a special lens cover to protect the surgeon's eye from back scatter.
- Using a smoke evacuator system during all laser surgery to absorb the plume from the laser.
- Changing the smoke-evacuation filters as recommended by the manufacturer.
- Wearing high-filtration masks that filter particulate matter of at least 0.3 or 0.1 µm.
- Having methods available to deal with the hazard of fire such as:
  - sterile water or normal saline on the set up to deal with a fire on or near the patient; or
  - a halon fire extinguisher immediately available to the laser theatre.
- Using non-reflective or ebonised instrumentation, and if non-reflective instruments are near the laser beam, then they should be covered with wet sponges.
- Not using alcoholic prep solutions or having combustible materials near where the laser beam is being used.

- Using wet or non-flammable drapes during the procedure and monitoring the wetness of the drapes throughout.
- Ensuring the surgeon identifies the laser foot pedal and maintains sole control of it.
- Using a commercially manufactured laser endotracheal tube during laser surgery to the oropharynx.[1]

The nurse who has been certified as the laser safety nurse during the procedure should be assigned to the laser and should not be involved in circulating/scouting duties during the procedure.

It is the responsibility of the hospital to ensure that all personnel using lasers receive the following.

- Proper training and credentials.
- Hold courses regularly to keep them current with new technology and procedures.
- Implement accredited policies and procedures to provide safe guidelines.
- Provide correct and adequate PPE.
- Establish a laser committee with suitable advisory personnel within the institution.
- Complete the appropriate documentation with each case.

LATEX ALLERGY

Andrea Thompson

Natural rubber latex is a product harvested from the rubber tree as a milky sap. It is valued for its strength, flexibility and durability in healthcare items such as surgical gloves, catheters, injectable bungs and stoppers on vials.

Safety measures

Because it is a natural product, latex contains proteins. Certain individuals when exposed to these proteins develop an allergy. Latex allergy affects perioperative nurses both through their occupational exposure to the allergen,[12] and because of the risk that some of our patients may experience a life-threatening reaction to latex products in the operating theatre.[13]

Particular groups have been identified as having a higher risk of developing a latex allergy.[14] Those with long-term exposure to the agent such as patients with chronic bladder catheterisations (spina bifida, spinal cord injuries, etc.) or those who have endured multiple operations are at much greater risk of developing antibodies to the latex proteins. Healthcare workers, with their daily exposure to latex products, and the rubber industry workers who collect and manufacture the raw product are also at a greater risk than the general population. Patients with a history of atopy and multiple allergies (especially certain fruit allergies, and a history of reactions after handling rubber balloons and other consumer items) are often at greater risk of latex allergy. Those patients who have had a previous unexplained anaphylaxis during surgery (not attributed to drugs) should be treated with caution.

Those affected by an allergy to latex may display a delayed or immediate reaction. A delayed reaction (type 4 cell-mediated allergic reaction) may occur hours or days after contact with latex products. The reaction is generally localised to the area of contact. For healthcare workers wearing gloves, this may lead to a contact dermatitis ranging from a mild skin irritation to rashes, itching, cracking and fissuring of the skin. Chronic skin changes such as thickening and scaling may occur.

An immediate allergic reaction (type 1 or anaphylactic reaction) occurs within minutes of exposure.[15] The reaction may be localised (tingling and swelling of the lips after contact with balloons, hives or eczema on contact with rubber household gloves or latex surgical gloves) or systemic (anaphylactic shock). Anaphylactic shock is an acute life-threatening event. When exposed to certain allergens, some people produce immunoglobulin E (IgE) antibodies that bind to the surface of mast cells and basophils. Whenever that individual is further exposed to the same allergen, it attaches to those IgE antibodies,

stimulating a chemical chain of events that leads to the anaphylactic reaction. The chemicals released cause vasodilation, increased capillary wall permeability, contraction of the smooth muscle of the airways and gut, and increased mucous secretion. The patient becomes tachycardic and hypotensive and may wheeze or, if intubated, show signs of bronchospasm. The skin becomes flushed and may develop hives or weals; facial oedema is most marked around the eyes and lips. Laryngeal oedema causes respiratory distress and makes intubation difficult. Complete circulatory collapse may occur.

When an anaphylactic reaction is suspected, the offending agent needs to be identified and removed. In the perioperative setting, when many drugs are often given in sequence, it can be difficult to isolate the offending agent. Reactions to latex can occur on induction or well into the surgery itself. A level of suspicion of latex allergy must always be maintained in the perioperative environment. Treatment of anaphylactic shock is intravenous adrenaline given in bolus form. The adrenaline dilates the airways, increases heart rate and contractility, and causes peripheral vasoconstriction.[15,16] Fluids are given to support the blood pressure, but the nurse needs to be aware that some colloid solutions contain latex in the bung. The airway is maintained by intubating and ventilating if necessary with 100% oxygen.

Avoidance of anaphylaxis in the latex-allergic patient involves careful questioning of all preoperative patients to ascertain those at risk. For patients with a known allergy, careful preparation of the perioperative environment is essential.[13] All latex items must be removed and replaced with latex-free alternatives. For items that do not have a latex-free alternative, consideration must be given to the necessity of the item, and, if possible, the item should be shielded from the patient. Each perioperative unit will have a latex policy outlining the steps to be taken. A list of products containing latex and their latex-free alternatives should also be kept with the policy. A special latex-free trolley or basket should be set up. All areas that will be looking after the patient must be made aware, in advance, of the allergy.

Perioperative staff are at a greater than average risk of developing a latex allergy.[17] With many staff members, this is in the form of a delayed reaction manifesting as changes to skin integrity. Affected staff should use non-latex gloves. The use of non-powdered gloves will decrease the level of airborne allergens. Staff showing signs of a latex allergy should see their manager to arrange for follow-up and testing. In extreme cases, transfer out of the perioperative unit may be necessary.

References

1. Meeker RH, Rothrock JC. *Alexander's Care of the Patient in Surgery*, 11th edn. St Louis: Mosby.
2. Adviser in Sterilizing Services. *Sterilizing Services Fact Sheet #5*. Brisbane: Communicable Diseases Unit, Queensland Health.
3. National Health and Occupational Safety Commission. *Exposure standards accepted December 1995: glutaraldehyde*. Canberra. Available from URL: http://www.worksafe.gov.au/databases/exp/az/Glutaraldehyde.htm
4. International Labour Organization, International Occupational Health and Safety Information Centre. *Glutaraldehyde*, 2000. Available from http://www.ilo.org/public/english/protection/safework/cis/products/icsc/dtasht/_icsc01/icsc0158.htm
5. Department of Health and Human Services USA, National Toxicology Program. *Chemical Health and Safety Data*, 2000. Available from URL: http://157.98.6.102/cgi/iH_Indexes/Chem_H&S/iH_Chem_H&S_Frames.html
6. *Worksafe Australia Hazard Alert No. 1*, October. Canberra: National Health and Occupational Safety Commission, 1991.
7. *Policy and Procedure Manual*. Brisbane: Princess Alexandra Hospital, 1999.
8. Wicker P. Electrosurgery in perioperative practice. *Br J Perioper Nurs* 2000; 10: 221–226.
9. Valleylab. *Principles of Electrosurgery*. Lane Cove: Tyco Healthcare Australia, 2000.
10. *Standards and Recommended Practices*. Denver: Association of Operating Room Nurses, 1993.
11. Fairchild SS. *Perioperative Nursing: Principles and Practice*, 2nd edn. Boston: Little, Brown, 1996.
12. Lopes MHB, Lopes RAM. Latex allergy in health care personnel. *AORN J* 2000; 72: 42–43, 45–46, 55–56.
13. Baumann NH. Latex allergy: an orthopaedic case presentation and considerations in patient care. *Orthop Nurs* 1999; 18: 15–22.
14. Bowyer RVS. Latex allergy: how to identify it and the people at risk. *J Clin Nurs* 1999; 8: 144–149.
15. Tortora GJ, Grabowski SR. *Principles of Anatomy and Physiology*. New York: HarperCollins, 1996.
16. Kaufman L, Taberner PV eds. *Pharmacology in the Practice of Anaesthesia*. London: Arnold, 1996.
17. Kim KT, Graves PB, Safadi GS, Alhadeff G, Metcalfe J. Implementation recommendations for making health care facilities latex safe. *AORN J* 1998; 67: 615–618, 621–624, 626.

6 | Patient positioning

Helen Werder and Maria Anderson

Helen Werder

Patient positioning is a team effort between the anaesthetist, nursing staff, operational officers and the surgeon. The patient should be positioned on the table to allow for maximum safety and comfort for the patient, for maximum access to the operative field for the surgeon, and to allow for maintenance of anaesthesia and observation by the anaesthetist. The patient should be positioned without compromise to respiratory and circulatory functions or neuromuscular structures. The optimal position may be achieved using appropriate positioning aids that will not obstruct or interfere with patient care.

Staff members involved in the positioning of patients should remember the following points before undertaking the procedure:

- Acquaint yourself beforehand with the mechanism of the operating table: raising, lowering, tilting and breaking of the parts.
- Assembly of all attachments to be used before the arrival of the patient.
- Be familiar with the various positions necessary to give the best access to the operative field.
- Placement of the patient in as comfortable a position as possible.
- Placement of the patient in the correct position when a 'break' in the table is needed intraoperatively.
- Prevention of any interference with the respiration of the patient whilst moving, e.g. pressure of the arms on the chest.
- Ensure the patient is fully anaesthetised before positioning.
- Never reposition the anaesthetised patient without supervision from the anaesthetist.

- Avoid flapping the linen whilst positioning as lint and bacteria thrown into the air may settle on the sterile field.
- Diathermy plate must be applied **after** the patient is positioned and rechecked if repositioning occurs.
- Registered nurse must check the diathermy plate for manufacturing flaws and the positioning of the plate before application.
- Table fittings must be placed so that there is no obstruction to the incision area for the surgeon during the operation.
- All fittings and attachments should be tightened so that no alteration of the patient's position can occur intraoperatively.
- Staff involved in moving the patient should protect themselves by observing good manual-handling techniques.

NURSING CONSIDERATIONS DURING POSITIONING

During the positioning of the patient on the operating table, the perioperative nurse should be aware of his/her responsibilities. These responsibilities include the following:

- Maintenance of unimpaired respiratory action throughout the procedure.
- Maintenance of physiological alignment with protection of muscles, nerves and bony prominences from pressure.
- Maintenance of adequate circulation avoiding direct peripheral pressures that affect venous return.
- Limiting of patient exposure to the area required for surgical/anaesthetic intervention thus maintaining patient dignity and temperature.

Patient positioning

- Explanation of all activities and rationale to the patient who will be conscious during the procedure and before induction to the patient receiving general anaesthesia.
- Avoidance of any part of the patient touching any metal part of the table.
- Need for sufficient staff and equipment for the positioning of the patient.
- Requirement that the scrub team does not lean on any part of the patient intraoperatively.

TABLE FEATURES FOR POSITIONING

Before attempting to position patients, the staff must practise to become familiar with the mechanisms of the different operating tables used in the operating rooms. Most modern tables consist of a rectangular metal top that rests upon a hydraulic, wheeled base. The table top is divided into two, three or four hinged sections, each of which can be manipulated by means of a manual lever or electronically see Fig 6.1. The individual sections of the table can be fixed or extended so that any desired position can be obtained. The joints of the table are called 'breaks' and the procedure of manipulating the sections is called 'breaking the table'. A cross bar between the two upper sections of the table can be used as a body elevator and is useful when gaining access to the gall bladder or kidney regions. Each table can be fitted with metal sockets (may be called 'knuckles') that slide on side rails to accommodate the insertion of different table attachments such as the stirrups or arm boards. Neurosurgical headrests or table extensions are detachable sections that can be used to replace foot or head sections for the appropriate surgical procedures. The entire table can be tilted

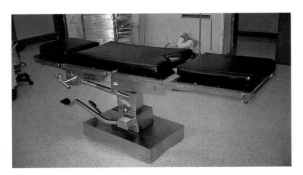

Fig. 6.1 Operating table

from side to side or raised and lowered dependent on the position required. The table has a wheel brake for stabilisation, which must always be applied when the table is in use.

SPECIAL EQUIPMENT AND TABLE ATTACHMENTS FOR POSITIONING

Operating table attachments and special equipment used in positioning are designed to stabilise the patient in the desired position, giving the best exposure of the operative area whilst providing safety and comfort. To facilitate this action further, all attachments must be adequately padded to prevent trauma to the patient.

Anaesthetic screen

This holds the sterile drapes away from the patient's face, separating the non-sterile area from the sterile field and permitting observation of the airway area by the anaesthetist. This may take the form of a metal bar or two or more intravenous stands and is used for all operations below the level of the head.

Armboard

This is used to support the arm not resting at the patient's side or across the chest. The anaesthetist for the purpose of intravenous therapy can request this position, or the arm's safety may be compromised by the position of the patient, e.g. hip operation, or for very obese patients where there is no space on the table beside them for their arms.

Stirrups

Stirrups are metal posts placed one on each side of the table at the lower break to support the legs and feet in the lithotomy position. The stirrups hold the foot and lower leg in a padded support, in good anatomical alignment and without pressure to the calf area of the lower leg. This type of support is preferable.

Lateral supports and body rests

Lateral supports are padded supports secured into the metal side rail sockets and positioned to support the chest and pelvic regions during surgery requiring a lateral position.

Pillows, gel-like horseshoes, doughnuts, sandbags and roll supports

These aids are used for stabilising the head and face or for providing support and protection to susceptible areas during surgery (see Fig. 6.2).

The positions for various operative procedures are described and shown in table 6.1 and Figs 6.3 to 6.10.

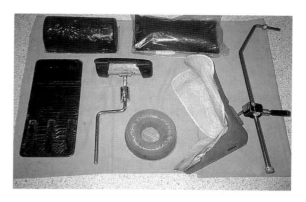

Fig. 6.2 Operating table accessories

Table 6.1 **Description of surgical positions and potential complications**

Table 6.1a
Supine/dorsal position

Position	Details to observe	Potential complications
Patient lies on back Arms placed by the side or on the patient's chest Arm may be placed on an armboard at an angle < 90° to the body Small pillow is placed under the head Legs are uncrossed with a small pad placed under the ankles to relieve pressure and to aid venous return Basic position may be modified for specific operations, e.g. plastic reconstructive operations	Head is not hyperextended Arm is not abducted beyond 90° Armboard is padded Hands on the armboards are supinated Arms do not overlap the table edge or hang over the edge Bony prominences are protected – occiput, scapulae, thoracic vertebrae, olecranon, sacrum and coccyx and calcaneus Pad under the ankles does not hyper-extend the legs Patient is protected from the metal of the bed	Backache may result from unsupported lumbosacral curvature Over abduction of the arm (> 90°) on the board may stretch the brachial plexus over the head of the humerus, resulting in paralysis of the arm and hand Elbow or arm hanging over the table may result in nerve palsy. Pressure on the elbow may result in ulnar palsy and if on the middle of the upper arm, a radial palsy may result Tight restraints on the wrist may result in peripheral nerve damage and on the humerus may result in radial nerve palsy Continuous pressure on the calves during long operations may cause venous stasis resulting in thrombosis that if detached has the potential for pulmonary embolus

Table 6.1b
Prone position

Position	Details to observe	Potential complications
Patient anaesthetised in the supine position and gently turned onto their abdomen Arms are placed at the side during movement of the patient Anaesthetist protects the airway and coordinates the positioning of the patient Movement of the anaesthetised patient must be gentle and slow Pillows are placed under the shoulders, hips and feet Arms may then be placed above the head Bridges or specially shaped supports may be used if spinal or lumbar surgery is being carried out This position is used for operations on all posterior sections of the body	Pillow or folded towels to be placed under shoulders and hips to allow free movement of the chest for respiration, reduction of pressure on the abdomen and inferior vena cava reducing venous oozing at the operation site Pillow under the feet Head is not hyperextended, placed on the side and is supported by a pillow or doughnut Potential pressure points are protected – cheek and ear, acromion process, breasts (women), genitalia (men), patella, dorsum of foot, toes	Lower neck and upper back pain can occur from hyperextension of the head Arm restrainers pressing on the ulnar nerve at the elbow or the radial nerve at the humerus can cause nerve palsies. Hypotension can result from pressure on the inferior vena cava, along with pooling of venous blood in the lower extremities Shoulder dislocation or brachial plexus injury can occur when placing arms over the patient's head Arms should be slowly lowered towards the floor and brought up in an arc while the elbow is flexed Arms should not be extended > 90°

Table 6.1c
Knee–chest position

Position	Details to observe	Potential complications
Patient anaesthetised in the supine position then turned into the prone position Legs are abducted and flexed together at right angles to the body with knees flexed and hips elevated Head, shoulders and chest rest on pillows on the table Arms are placed above the head Pillows, foam pads, supports and tape are used to stabilise the patient. A padded bracket is used to support the buttocks This position is mainly used for spinal surgery	Legs are moved together to prevent back strain Arms are gently placed in the position above the head as in a prone position The buttock-supporting bracket is placed so that the seat is supporting the ischial tuberosities not the femoral shafts Bracket is well padded and the attachment to the table is well tightened Head is not hyperextended and placed to the side on a pillow or doughnut Bony prominences and potential pressure points are protected – cheek and ear (head on side), forehead, eyes and nose (head face down), acromion process, breasts (women), genitalia (men), patella, dorsum of feet, toes	Lower neck and upper back pain can occur from hyperextension of the head Arm restrainers pressing on the ulnar nerve at the elbow or the radial nerve at the humerus can cause nerve palsies Hypotension can result from pressure on the inferior vena cava, along with pooling of venous blood in the lower extremities Shoulder dislocation or brachial plexus injury can occur when placing arms over the patient's head Arms should be slowly lowered towards the floor and brought up in an arc while the elbow is flexed Arms should not be extended > 90° Patient may fall from the table if brackets are not secure and fail to support the patient's weight

Table 6.1d
Kidney/lateral position

Position	Details to observe	Potential complications
Patient is anaesthetised in the supine and then gently turned with the side to be operated on upper-most and their back near the edge of the table Pillow is placed between the legs with the lower leg flexed to 90° and the upper leg nearly straight Upper arm is supported in an arm-rest or on a pillow and the lower arm remains on the mattress and flexed near the face or is placed on an arm board For kidney procedures, the patient is positioned so that the iliac crest is level with the centre break of the table Table is flexed so the operative area is horizontal. A kidney rest may also be raised to increase exposure and access Lateral position is maintained by the use of sandbags or two kidney supporting braces attached to the sides of the table. The short brace is to the back as it is closest to the table edge and the long brace attaches in front of the patient Head is supported on a pillow This position is used for kidney or chest operations	If the kidney rest or table break is used, it must be correctly level with the iliac crest to prevent interference with respiration and severe postoperative backache Head is supported on a headrest or pillow ensuring the ear is not trapped Arms are supported by padded arm-rests, arm boards and/or pillows Both legs are protected with padding, especially the down leg of the patient Bony prominences are protected – acromion process, ribs, iliac crest, greater trochanter, medial and lateral femoral epicondyles and tibial condyles, malleolus	If kidney rest is raised too much, it can cause cyanosis due to difficulty in expanding the lungs Also, interference with the return of the blood to the heart can cause a serious fall in blood pressure Injuries to the brachial plexus, median, radial and ulnar nerves can occur if the upper arm is not supported. Stretching of the brachial plexus can occur if the head is not fully supported. Damage can occur to the perineal nerve from compression on the down knee against a hard surface.

Patient positioning

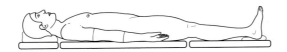

Fig. 6.3 Surgical positions and potential complications: supine

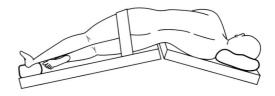

Fig. 6.6 Surgical positions and potential complications: kidney lateral

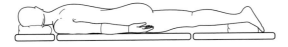

Fig. 6.4 Surgical positions and potential complications: prone

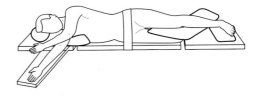

Fig. 6.7 Surgical positions and potential complications: lateral

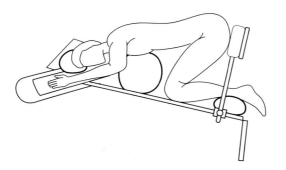

Fig. 6.5 Surgical positions and potential complications: knee chest position

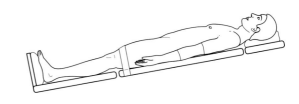

Fig. 6.8 Surgical positions and potential complications: reverse Trendelenburg

SUMMARY OF COMPLICATIONS FROM POOR POSITIONING

Pressure on nerves

Nerves can be damaged by pressure or by stretching. The most common nerves affected during positioning of the patient are the following.

- **Brachial plexus**: can be damaged by extreme abduction of the arm on an armboard, the head not being supported when in the lateral position and the arms being over extended above the head when in the prone position.

- **Radial nerve**: can be damaged by the upper part of the arm hanging over the table edge or by a projection on the table pressing against the humerus.
- **Ulnar nerve**: can be damaged by the elbow hanging over the edge of the table.
- **Common peroneal nerve**: can be damaged and foot drop can occur by pressure being placed on the leg at the knee in the lateral and lithotomy positions.
- **Tibial nerve**: can be damaged when the legs are crossed for prolonged periods.
- **Peripheral nerves**: can be damaged by over tight strapping of the arm onto the armboard.

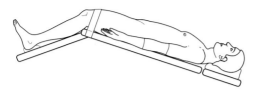

Fig. 6.9 Surgical positions and potential complications: Trendelenburg

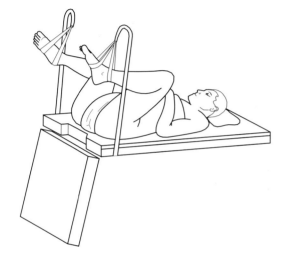

Fig. 6.10 Surgical positions and potential complications: lithotomy

Pressure on veins

Continuous pressure on the calves may cause venous stasis during long operations with the patient in the supine position. This stasis may cause thrombosis and a portion of the thrombus may become detached resulting in pulmonary embolus. Crossing of the legs causes compression of the small saphenous vein of the upper leg and small and long saphenous veins and dorsalis pedis artery of the lower leg. These actions further contribute to venous stasis.

Vascular damage

Accompanying brachial plexus injury may be the obliteration of the radial pulse resultant from the over extension of the arm causing compression on the subclavian artery between the clavicle and the first rib.

Muscle and ligament strain

Muscles and ligaments are potentially subject to strains caused by poor positioning and movement. The most common strains are the following.

- Backache caused by an unsupported lumbosacral curve in the supine position.
- Backache caused when legs are not raised and lowered together into the lithotomy position.
- Backache caused by incorrect positioning of the kidney rest/table break in the lateral position.
- Lower neck and upper back pain caused by hyperextension of the head in the prone position.
- Shoulder strain caused by insufficient support or poor technique when positioning the arms over the patient's head in the prone position.

Skin pressure

Decubitus ulcers can develop as a consequence of poor positioning and inadequate protection. The main contributing factors that place patients at high risk of ulcer formation are age, an underlying medical condition, general health and nutritional status, and the duration the pressure is sustained. The duration rather than intensity is believed to be the most crucial contributing factor in ulcer development.

All bony prominences where pressure is applied may be affected and should be protected.

Protection from metal

The patient should have no part of their anatomy touching the metal parts of the operating table as diathermy burn can result if the current earths itself via this pathway.

POSITIONING THE ELDERLY PATIENT

Positioning of the elderly patient for surgery requires additional care and consideration from the operative team as they have fragile skin, arthritic joints, a limited range of motion or even paralysis.[1-3] The major challenge is to preserve and protect the skin integrity of the surgical patient. Loss of subcutaneous fat and decreased peripheral circulation increase elderly patients' risks for decubitus ulcers especially when they undergo prolonged immobility and pressure. Poor skin turgor, tissue fragility and ageing changes in the skin accentuate bony prominences and care must be taken to avoid shearing injuries when moving and positioning the elderly patient. Lifting the patient where possible, rather than sliding or dragging, can facilitate this. The use of tape to secure elderly patients' limbs or tubes should be avoided as tape can tear fragile skin.

Intraoperatively, bony prominences should be well protected, supported and padded to avoid pressure on these places.[4] Lack of mobility of the elderly patient can tend to difficulty in positioning of the limbs and to muscular strains unrelated to the operative site postoperatively. Musculoskeletal deformity or restriction may mean the elderly patient cannot fully extend the spine, neck or upper and lower extremities.[2] The use of pillows or padding devices can compensate for these restrictions and where possible the patients should be allowed to position themselves for maximum comfort before anaesthesia. This will decrease the likelihood of fractures or joint strains and postoperative pain.

CHILDREN

Maria Anderson

Children are at the same risk of injury from poor positioning as adults, so the same care must be given. Care should be taken to protect the child from injury at all times in the OR, from their admission to the OR suite, during anaesthesia induction, throughout the operation and in the Post-Anaesthesia Care Unit.

Children react to drugs in ways that are sometimes different to adults, or may be much more rapid. Anaesthetic induction and recovery may be fast so children must never be left unattended at any time while in the OR.

When positioning children it is important to think of 'appropriate size'. Common sense dictates that you would not give a child or an infant the same size pillow as an adult would use. Select the right size

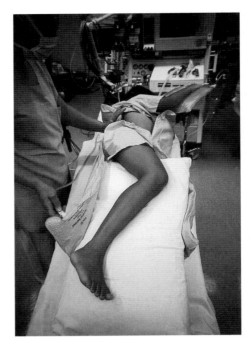

Fig. 6.11 Evacuatable mattress

extras or attachments to ensure the optimal safety for your patient.

An evacuatable mattress filled with polystyrene balls is sometimes used with children. The patient is positioned on the mattress, which is then pushed into place. A suction unit is attached, air is extracted and the mattress fits securely around the child. It may be necessary to use safety straps to stabilise the patient fully.

Because infants lose body heat rapidly and small babies are physiologically incapable of maintaining their body heat efficiently, a heating mattress is always used. For long operations, a heating unit that blows hot air onto the patient can be used, and limbs and exposed areas in small babies are wrapped in cotton wool. The temperature of the OR is increased if an infant is the patient.

Positions for surgery in paediatrics

Basic positions as listed for adults are used in paediatrics. However, there are some modifications. Children are easier to move and their joints much more pliable than those of adults. However, care must be taken not to overextend limbs or to keep a child in one position for long periods. While their circulation is faster than adults' and less at risk of thromboses, these do occur. Because of the small volume of organs such as the lungs, children are often more rapidly physiologically compromised. Constant observation of vital signs is imperative as children can become distressed very rapidly.

Some positions not listed in the adults' section are given in the following.

- Boyle Davis gag position for adenotonsillectomy: the mouth gag and tongue depressor is combined and supported by metal suspension rods to give a clear view and good access to the oral cavity. The child's head is hyperextended back and the neck supported by a sandbag and head ring.
- Position for microlaryngeal surgery with the use of the laryngoscopy support bar: the microlaryngoscope is placed into the oropharynx, which is then supported by the Benjamin Parsons stabiliser, which is subsequently placed on the microlaryngoscopy support tray, thus allowing the surgeon the freedom to use both hands for the procedure. The support tray is attached to the table and sits just above the patient's chest.
- Children sometimes require the application of a hip spica after operations such as correction of congenital abnormalities of the hips, postfemoral osteotomy surgery and repair of fractured femur. There are several devices that are in use for this application. To use the hip spica-positioning box effectively, there must be enough staff to support and maintain stability of the child.

References

1. Kaczmarowski N. *Patient Care in the Operating Room*. Melbourne: Churchill Livingstone, 1982.
2. Meeker RH, Rothrock JC. *Alexander's Care of the Patient in Surgery*, 11th edn. St Louis: Mosby, 1995.
3. Lusis SA. The challenges of nursing elderly surgical patients. *AORN J* 1996; 64: 954–955, 957–962.
4. Fairchild SS. *Perioperative Nursing: Principles and Practice*, 2nd edn. Boston: Little, Brown, 1996.

Perioperative care of
the adult patient

7 | Anaesthesia

Andrea M. Thompson

PATIENT UNDERGOING ANAESTHESIA

The patient undergoing an operation will undergo anaesthesia – be it a local, regional or general anaesthetic. The anaesthetic nurse's role is to provide continuing care to the patient during their operative experience. The anaesthetic nurse does this by providing individualised care appropriate to each patient's pre-existing medical conditions, their age, psychological status and the type of surgery and anaesthetic the patient will encounter. In addition to the nurse's existing nursing skills and knowledge, the anaesthetic nurse has an understanding of anaesthetic drugs, equipment, techniques and critical events. All aspects of the anaesthetic nurse's role – direct patient care and maintenance of equipment – aim to protect the physiological and psychological safety of the patient.

ANAESTHETIC NURSE'S ROLE

The role of the anaesthetic nurse is to ensure the physical and psychological safety of the patient undergoing anaesthesia. The anaesthetic nurse provides continuity of the patient's general nursing care into the perioperative environment. The anaesthetic nurse works together with the anaesthetist to ensure optimal patient outcomes. Other duties of the anaesthetic nurse are the following:

- Checking of anaesthetic machine, monitors and ancillary equipment.
- Assessment and preparation of patient-specific equipment and monitors.
- Checking in of patients on arrival to theatre.
- Assessing the patient for anxiety, the effect of premedication and the understanding of events.
- Continued care and observance of the patient in the anaesthetic holding area or room.
- Attachment and assessment of monitoring devices.
- Assistance with regional anaesthesia procedures.
- Assistance with general anaesthesia: induction, maintenance and emergence.
- Assisting with the insertion of infusion and invasive monitoring lines.
- Maintenance of patient documentation.
- Assist with patient transfers, positioning and pressure care.
- Maintaining normothermia of the patient.
- Prepare and administer drug infusions, antibiotics, etc.
- Transfer and handover to post anaesthesia care or Intensive Care Unit staff.

The role of the anaesthetic nurse may vary between institutions and countries. In the USA, nurses can undergo further study to become nurse anaesthetists, independent practitioners who administer anaesthetics. In smaller hospitals, the anaesthetic nurse may rotate through the scout, scrub and recovery roles. In large tertiary-level hospitals, the anaesthetic nurse is often a specialist practitioner with postgraduate qualifications. Anaesthetic technicians replace nurses in some institutions, fulfilling many of the technical duties incorporated in the role.

ANAESTHESIA

For centuries, man has tried to ease pain and later facilitate surgeries. Alcohol, poultices, herbs and opium have been used with varying degrees of success. Early surgery was swift and brutal, the patients experiencing excruciating pain. The era of modern anaesthesia was heralded in 1846 when

Anaesthesia

William Morton first demonstrated surgical anaesthesia using ether.[1]

'Anaesthesia' is an ancient Greek word meaning 'not or without sensation'. It aptly describes what anaesthesia still is today. Anaesthesia facilitates surgery by removing the sensation of pain and its associated reflex responses. Safe anaesthesia involves the control and maintenance of homeostasis, control and maintenance of the airway and tissue oxygenation, adequate blood pressure and organ perfusion, maintenance of circulating volume, temperature control, and protection of the anaesthetised body. This may require management of serious concurrent disease states or the treatment of injury-related shock.

Anaesthetics can be described as general or regional. In general anaesthesia, the patient is rendered unconscious and may or may not be muscle paralysed. In regional anaesthesia, the operative site is anaesthetised using either a block technique or local infiltration. Sedation may be given. The anaesthetic technique is decided upon by the anaesthetist having assessed the type and duration of surgery, the patient's medical status and the patient's wishes.

PREOPERATIVE ASSESSMENT

Before any operation, the anaesthetist will assess the patient's medical suitability to undergo anaesthesia. This may occur in a preadmission clinic, where the patient is seen, assessed and their anaesthesia discussed before their hospital admission date. This is an effective way of screening elective patients and ensuring their medical status is optimised well before their surgery time. Any relevant tests or X-rays can be ordered and performed. With patients often coming into hospital on the day of surgery, it ensures that any pre-existing concerns are noted, and gives the patient the opportunity to discuss their anaesthetic in a more relaxed environment. Many institutions ask patients to complete a preanaesthetic questionnaire before being seen by the anaesthetist (Fig 7.1). This gives patients time to ensure the completeness of their responses, and guides the anaesthetist to any areas of concern. Urgency of operation will dictate the timing and extent of the preoperative assessment in emergency cases.

The preanaesthesia assessment will include information about the patient's current state of health. Any health concerns and medications are discussed and assessed for their impact on the patient's ability to undergo anaesthesia. The patient is asked about any cardiac, renal, hepatic, endocrine, respiratory or central nervous system symptoms or disease. The patient's intake of tobacco, alcohol or illicit drugs is questioned. Has the patient had any previous anaesthetics, and were there any problems? Has anyone in the patient's family had any problems with anaesthesia? Does the patient have any drug allergies? Does the patient have gastric reflux? All of these answers are evaluated and guide the anaesthetist in deciding the most appropriate type of anaesthesia. The airway is checked with relation to ease of intubation. The heart and lungs are auscultated with a stethoscope. The patient's medical chart and records of any previous anaesthetics are read. The anaesthetist will also check the patient's relevant blood tests, and if the patient is over 50 years of age, the electrocardiograph (ECG) and chest X-ray are used, and specialist testing, e.g. cardiac function, may be required for some patients.

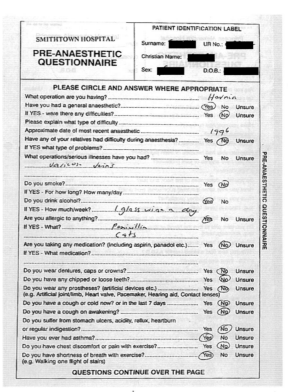

Fig. 7.1 Preanaesthetic questionnaire

ASA status

After thorough assessment of the patient's medical condition, the anaesthetist will give the patient an ASA rating.[2,3] The American Society of Anaesthesiologists devised the rating to enable anaesthetists to class patients according to existing medical status and therefore to assess their anaesthetic risk. Perioperative mortality rates increase in relation to the ASA rating (Table 7.1).

The anaesthetic nurse will also assess the patient, usually on their arrival in the operating suite. The nurse assesses the patient's mental status, anxiety levels and understanding of the operative experience, as well as their physical status. The presence and patency of intravenous (IV) cannulas, infusions, urinary catheters, drains or any other therapeutic device is checked. The patient's general condition is noted, and the nurse will base the need for interventions on this. Often the patient will mention to the nurse information pertinent to the anaesthetic, and this should be shared with the anaesthetist.

ANAESTHETIC EQUIPMENT

ANAESTHETIC MACHINE

The purpose of an anaesthetic machine is to deliver gases and vapours, at set concentrations, to the patient. It combines the properties needed to do this into a functional design that incorporates room for monitoring and ventilation systems and provides an area used as a workstation. Newer electronic models may include in-built monitors and ventilators. For practical purposes, anaesthetic machines must be sturdy, movable and have storage space for ancillary equipment such as facemasks, laryngoscopes and other supplies.

Flow of gases

Gas supplies (oxygen, nitrous oxide and medial air) enter the anaesthetic machine from either the piped bulk gas supply or from attached cylinders. Pressure regulators inside the machine decrease the pressure of the gases to a level safe for delivery to the patient. Flowmeters allow regulation of the flow of gas to the patient. One flowmeter for each gas is supplied (1 in Fig 7.2) . Vaporisers (2 in Fig 7.2) turn the liquid anaesthetic agent into a vapour, which is added to the gas supplied to the patient by dialling up the required percentage. Gases and vapour at the preset concentrations are delivered at a common gas outlet (3 in Fig 7.2). The chosen breathing system is connected to the standardised connector. Internal safety features include an oxygen failure device that detects falling pressure of the supplied oxygen. It alarms audibly and, in some machines, visually. It cuts off the nitrous oxide supply to the patient. An antihypoxia device is incorporated into flowmeters to prevent the inadvertent delivery of an hypoxic mix of gases to the patient. The nitrous oxide will not flow unless there is at least 25% of oxygen dialled up. An emergency oxygen button (4 in Fig 7.2) delivers high-flow and pressure oxygen directly to the common gas outlet, bypassing flowmeters and vaporisers. The scavenging system removes gases and vapours vented from the breathing system to prevent contamination of the operating theatre. Low-pressure suction is used for this.

Equipment added to the anaesthetic machine

Suction (5 in Fig 7.2) is used to remove secretions and other contaminants from the airway. Ventilators (6 in Fig 7.2) automatically ventilate the lungs of the paralysed patient using positive pressure. They deliver a set volume to the patient at a set rate, with an expiratory pause to allow for passive exhalation. Gauges indicate the pressure levels during the ventilator cycle. High pressure can be generated if the volume

---

Table 7.1
ASA ratings[2]

1. Healthy
2. Mild systemic disease with no functional impairment
3. Moderate systemic disease with functional impairment
4. Severe systemic disease that is a constant threat to life
5. Not expected to survive 24 hours with or without surgery
6. Brain dead organ donor

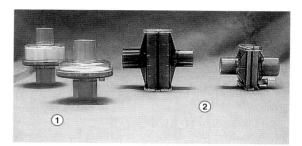

Fig. 7.4 Breathing system additions. 1. Filters. 2. Heat/moisture exchangers

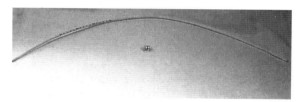

Fig. 7.5 Tube exchangers: placed through the *in situ* tube. The tube is removed and a new tube passed over the exchanger. A standard connector can be used to oxygenate the patient with the tube exchanger *in situ*. It is useful if reintubation is expected to be difficult

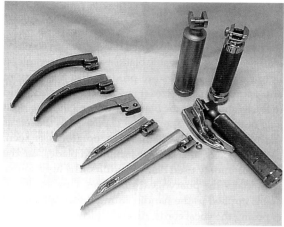

Fig. 7.7 Laryngoscopes

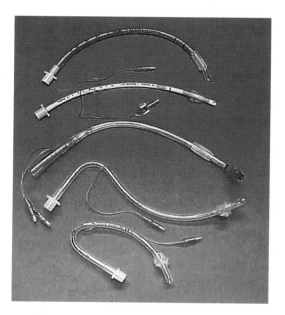

Fig. 7.8 Endotracheal tubes (ETT) Specialist tubes. Top to bottom: Reinforced, MLT, double lumen, nasal rae and oral rae

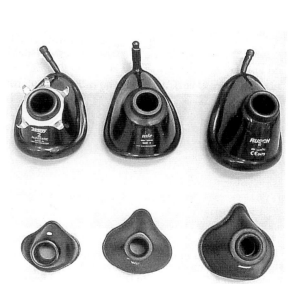

Fig. 7.6 Anaesthetic facemasks

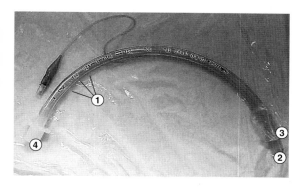

Fig. 7.9 Endotracheal tube. 1. Distance markings from the tip of the tube. 2. The bevel on the tip of the tube is designed to be atraumatic to tissues. 3. 'Murphy's eye' an extra hole on the side of the tube just above the tip 4. The standard 15mm connector.

protects the airway from contamination. In long-term intubation, cuff pressures are checked as high pressures against the tracheal wall can cause damage. Cuff designs and pressures vary between tubes and are selected on the proposed usage of the tube (long- or short-term).

Sometimes paediatric tubes are uncuffed. In children, the narrowest part of the airway is below the level of the vocal cords – this provides a natural seal.

Airways

Airways are used to maintain a patent airway by compensating for the decreased muscle tone and subsequent airway collapse and obstruction by the tongue or pharynx that occurs in the unconscious patient. Oropharyngeal airway (also called geudels airway) is inserted upside down and rotated through 180°. The nasopharyngeal airway is better tolerated during light anaesthesia or recovery. Airways are lubricated and inserted perpendicular to the plane of the face (Fig. 7.11)

The laryngeal mask airway (Fig 7.12) sits above the level of the vocal cords to maintain a patent airway. It is most commonly used in spontaneously breathing anaesthetised patients, although positive pressure ventilation may be applied. The mask is used in operations where muscle relaxation is not required, where duration is less than 3 hours. It is not used in patients at risk of gastric reflux as the mask does not give complete protection against aspiration. It is reusable and comes in a range of adult and paediatric sizes.

For more airway equipment and explanation see Figures 7.13-15 below.

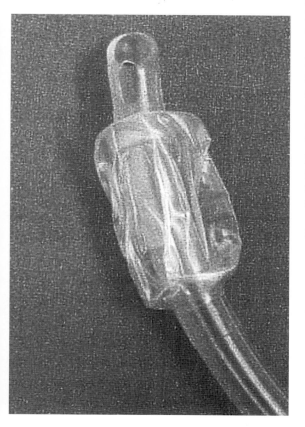

Fig. 7.10 Cuffs on endotracheal tubes

Anaesthesia

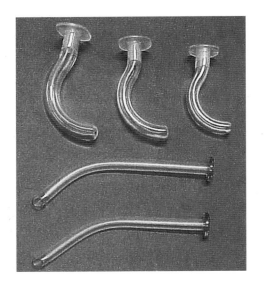

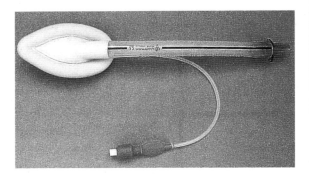

Fig. 7.11 Airways

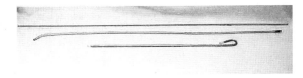

Fig. 7.14 **Introducers:** assist in the placement of the endotracheal tube (ETT). **Metal introducers:** inserted into the tube before intubation. They make the tube more rigid and can be used to alter the shape to suit the anatomy. **Gum elastic bougie:** inserted through the vocal cords under laryngoscope guidance; the ETT is then passed over the bougie. It is useful in difficult intubations when the larynx cannot be fully visualised

Fig. 7.12 Laryngeal mask airway

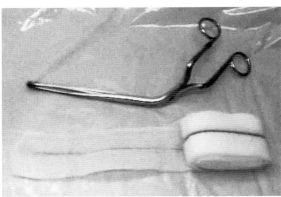

Fig. 7.15 **Magill's forceps and throat pack:** the forceps can be used to guide the tube through the larynx or to introduce a nasogastric tube or throat pack. It is used to remove foreign objects from the upper airway. A throat pack is a radio-opaque gauze pack placed into the pharynx above the vocal cords in the intubated patient. It collects blood and debris during operations on the nose or mouth to prevent it pooling above the tube cuff or contaminating the airway

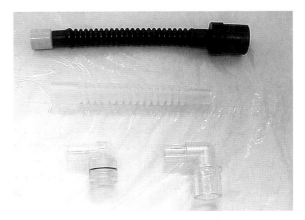

Fig. 7.13 **Liquorice sticks and elbow connectors:** connect the breathing circuit to the mask, endotracheal tube or laryngeal mask airway

GENERAL ANAESTHESIA

Under general anaesthesia, the patient is rendered unconscious. The aim of general anaesthesia is to provide a balance of hypnosis (sleep), muscle relaxation and analgesia. Reflexes are lost, including the response to the stimulus of surgery, and the protective reflexes of maintaining a patent airway. Maintenance of vital function comes under control of the anaesthetic personnel.

Table 7.2
Common IV induction agents

Name	Effects	Side-effects	Other
Thiopentone	sedation, hypnosis, anaesthesia; rapid onset, duration about 5 min	cardiac and respiratory depression; peripheral vasodilatation; pain on injection; anaphylaxis	powerful anticonvulsant; intra-arterial injection causes tissue damage; not used in porphyria patients; decreases cerebral O_2 consumption
Propofol	as for above	pain on injection; rapid injection may cause hypotension; involuntary movement can occur on induction; cardiac and respiratory depression	rapid recovery of consciousness; patients often experience pleasant dreams; can be used for maintenance of anaesthesia – TIVA (total intravenous anaesthesia), sedation during surgery or in ICU; dissolved in intra-lipid so beware of egg allergies
Methohexitone	as for above, more rapid awakening than thiopentone	cardiac and respiratory depression; involuntary muscle movement; pain on injection	lowers the seizure threshold – not for use in epileptics, but useful during ECT
Ketamine	produces 'dissociative anaesthesia'; anaesthesia occurs in 30–60 s, lasts 10–15 min; potent analgesic; bronchodilator	delirium, nightmares and hallucinations during recovery phase – avoid stimuli; increased heart rate and blood pressure; increased intracranial pressure; excessive salivation	used in the shocked patient because it increases heart rate and blood pressure; used in developing countries and at accident sites where equipment is limited; in lower doses, its analgesic properties are useful in palliative care; may be used in severe asthma

DRUGS USED IN GENERAL ANAESTHESIA

Premedication drugs

The administration of drugs before the patient's arrival in theatre

The aims of premedication drugs are varied. The most commonly given premedications include drugs to relieve anxiety and provide some sedation, and drugs to prevent nausea. Other drugs are given to prevent unwanted effects, such as excessive secretions or bronchospasm. Some types of drugs are given to increase patient safety, such as those designed to decrease gastric acidity. Analgesics may be given to provide pain relief, sedation and to decrease anxiety. The anaesthetist will also decide which of the patient's regular medications to continue preoperatively.

Induction agents

Induction agents transform the patient from the conscious to the unconscious state. They can be given intravenously or by the inhalational route. Inhalational induction agents include halothane and sevoflurane (Table 7.2).

Muscle relaxants

Muscle relaxants facilitate intubation and ventilation by paralysing the vocal cords and muscles of respira-

Anaesthesia

tion. They allow surgical access, especially abdominal, by relaxing muscles and stop reflex muscle contractions resulting from surgical stimuli.

Depolarising muscle relaxants

Suxamethonium is the only depolarising muscle relaxant in common use today. Paralysis occurs in less than 30 seconds after the patient fasciculates (twitches). Suxamethonium is broken down by plasma pseudocholinesterase, a naturally occuring enzyme in the blood, and duration of action is 3–5 minutes. It is used when there is a need for rapid onset of paralysis for intubation (full stomach) or if there is a need for rapid offset of paralysis (difficult intubations, short cases).

Side-effects can include:

- A small percentage of the population has altered or deficient plasma pseudocholinesterase – this causes prolonged paralysis.
- Potassium release: hyperkalaemia can result especially in patients with extensive burns or muscle damage, spinal injury or neuropathy, or renal failure.
- Raises intracranial and intraocular pressures.
- Causes postoperative muscle pains, especially in younger patients.
- Is a trigger for malignant hyperthermia.

Non-depolarising muscle relaxants

These block impulse receptor sites on the muscle. When more than 70% of these sites are occupied, paralysis occurs, usually within 3 minutes. Repeated boluses may be given intraoperatively to maintain paralysis, or an infusion may be run. Most are metabolised by the liver, and as the drug is cleared, muscle movement returns. Reversal of block can be increased by the use of an antagonist anticholinesterase drug (neostigmine). Atropine or glycopyrrolate are given with the anticholinesterase to prevent bradycardia (See Table 7.3).

Volatile anaesthetic agents

- Liquids made gaseous and delivered into the breathing system via calibrated vaporisers.
- Pass from the alveoli into the circulation.
- Used predominantly for maintenance of anaesthesia. May be used for induction, especially in children, with the difficult airway or in the needle phobic patient.

All volatile anaesthetic agents cause some dose-dependent degree of vasodilatation (with a resultant decrease in blood pressure), muscle relaxation (especially uterine) and respiratory depression. Volatile agents are potent anaesthetics, but have few analgesic properties. Dosage of the volatile agent is dialled on the vaporiser and is represented as a percentage of the fresh gas flow (see Table 7.4).

Nitrous oxide

Nitrous oxide is a colourless sweet-smelling gas that has potent analgesic qualities, but it is a weak anaesthetic. It is often used in combination with the volatile agents. For pain relief during labour or procedures, a premixed nitrous oxide–oxygen 1:1 mix called Entonox/Nitronox™ may be administered. In anaesthesia, the flow rate is controlled via the rotameters, where it is added to the fresh gas flow. Nitrous oxide is always administered with more than 25% oxygen to avoid hypoxia. Nitrous oxide diffuses into air-containing spaces within the body, expanding them. It will cause an increase in the size of a pneumothorax and causes bowel distension. When using an endotracheal tube with an air-filled cuff, nitrous oxide will diffuse into the cuff, causing an increase in pressure. Prolonged or repeated exposure to nitrous oxide inhibits vitamin B_{12} synthesis, causes bone marrow aplasia, anaemia and peripheral neuropathy. Diffusion hypoxia occurs at the end of the anaesthetic as nitrous oxide diffuses back into the alveoli, diluting the oxygen concentration. It is a transient effect and is treated by giving supplementary oxygen for the first 10 minutes postoperatively.

Narcotics

- Used to provide strong analgesia pre-, intra- and postoperatively.
- Intraoperatively given intravenously, may be administered orally, intramuscularly, subcutaneously, by IV bolus or infusion, by the epidural or spinal route.
- In large doses can be used to induce and maintain anaesthesia.
- Common side-effects include respiratory depression, sedation, nausea and vomiting.

Table 7.3
Paralysing agents

Name	Duration (min)	Side-effects	Other
Mivacurium	~15–20		metabolised by plasma pseudocholinesterase
Atracurium	~20	histamine release; hypotension	metabolised by Hoffman elimination – degrades at normal body temperature and pH
Cisatracurium	~20		less histamine release than atracurium
Vecuronium	~20		metabolised by the liver
Rocuronium	~20		rapid onset with large doses
Pancuronium	30–40	tachycardia, hypertension	steroid derivative; minimal histamine release

Table 7.4
Volatile anaesthetic agents

Agent	Advantages	Disadvantages
Ethrane		contraindicated in epileptics – can cause EEG changes in higher doses
Halothane	pleasant odour – useful for induction; non-irritant to airways; good bronchodilator	slowest onset and offset; trigger for malignant hyperthermia; precipitates arrhythmias with high levels of CO_2, or adrenaline; implicated in 'halothane hepatitis' after repeated doses; can cause postoperative shivering
Isoflurane	rapid onset – moderate offset; minimal cerebral blood flow changes – good for neurosurgery; minimal liver metabolism	pungent odour and airway irritation – not good for induction
Sevoflurane	rapid onset and offset – good for induction, fast waking; pleasant odour; minimal liver metabolism	may react with soda lime at low fresh gas flow rates

ANAESTHETIC TECHNIQUES

PREPARING FOR ANAESTHESIA

Adequate preparation of both the patient and anaesthetic equipment and resources is essential to the provision of safe anaesthetic care.

Patient preparation

- Preoperative assessment and routine tests.
- Optimisation of medical conditions: asthma, cardiac function, etc.
- Explanation of anaesthesia types, risks and procedures.
- Preoperative education: postoperative breathing exercises, deep vein thrombosis (DVT) prophylaxis.
- Fasting: the unconscious patient is at risk of regurgitation and aspiration as protective airway reflexes are lost. To minimise this risk, the patient is fasted before all elective surgery. This ensures the stomach is emptied of all food and drink before the patient is placed under general anaesthesia. Fasting times are based on the amount of time it takes food or drink to be passed from the stomach into the small intestine. Food-transit time is approximately 6 hours and clear fluid 2–4 hours. To ensure compliance and avoid confusion, patients are generally requested to withhold all oral intake from midnight before morning surgery, and from 6 a.m. for afternoon operations. Paediatric fasting times vary – older children can tolerate fasting more than neonates who may require regular or glucose feeds until 2 hours before surgery.

  Neutralisation of gastric acids – patients with a history of reflux or hiatus hernia may be given medication to decrease gastric acid production or to neutralise the acidity of the gastric contents.
- Regular medications: anaesthetists' or standing orders apply on which regular medication to give before surgery. Oral hypoglycaemics are withheld, insulin orders will be reviewed and perhaps changed to a sliding-scale dosage, coupled with a glucose infusion. Antihypertensives are generally administered, along with antiarrhythmics.
- Premedications are given as charted.
- Patient hygiene and theatre attire are as per institution policy.

- Communication aids: hearing aids and spectacles are best left with the patient to aid communication and prevent confusion and anxiety. Patients with language barriers or sensory impairments may require the assistance of an interpreter.
- Dentures: properly fitting dentures aid mask ventilation of the unconscious patient. Conversely, poorly fitting dentures can cause airway obstruction. Generally, dentures are removed before intubation. Each institution will have its own policy on dentures.
- Loose teeth in children should be noted on the preoperative checklist.
- Make-up and nail polish: should be removed for patient safety reasons. Make-up can obscure signs of cyanosis. Nail polish and artificial nails interfere with oximetry readings.

Anaesthetic preparation

- Anaesthetic machine is checked and functioning correctly.
- Monitoring equipment is present and functioning. Additional monitors as required are added.
- Airway equipment has been checked. The equipment required for this patient is prepared.
- IV lines and cannulation equipment is prepared.
- Additional invasive lines – if required the equipment is available.
- Pressure-relieving devices are ready if required.
- Warming equipment is available if needed.
- Equipment for regional techniques as required.
- Any other patient-specific needs are met.

ARRIVAL IN THEATRE COMPLEX

Anaesthetic considerations

- Checklist completed. Special note is made of fasting times and drug allergies.
- Premedication order is checked. Was the drug(s) given? What type of drug(s)? Expected effects – are they present?
- Have required regular medications been given?
- Anaesthetic nurse assessment.
- Patient is assessed for comfort and anxiety levels. Additional blankets may be required to compensate for the air-conditioning. Patients often

feel vulnerable lying flat on their trolleys – raising the head of the trolley may increase a patient's feeling of control. Anxiety levels are often minimised by the presence of friendly competent staff offering appropriate explanations of events.

The patient is taken to the operating room (OR), to a general holding bay or to an anaesthetic room adjacent to the operating theatre. An IV line is inserted and the patient may be given medication to sedate and calm them. Careful observation of the patient is necessary, as respiratory depression or other side-effects may occur. Regional anaesthetic techniques or the insertion of additional invasive lines may be undertaken in this area, and the anaesthetic nurse assists as required.

Parents are often encouraged to accompany their child to the OR and stay until the child is unconscious.[4] This requires education of the parent about how the child will look and feel as he/she becomes unconscious, and a nurse to accompany the parent and escort them from the theatre.

Into the theatre

The anaesthetic nurse assists with the safe transfer of the patient from the trolley to the operating table. Positioning is of great importance – special care is taken of nerves and bony prominences to prevent damage. Monitors are placed – oximetry, blood pressure cuff and ECG electrodes – taking care not to expose the awake patient. Oxygen will be given via the anaesthetic circuit before the induction of anaesthesia. Giving 100% oxygen before induction increases the oxygen reserves of the lungs.

Induction

Induction is the process of rendering the conscious, aware patient unconscious. Induction agents may be introduced intravenously, or the patient may breathe in the agent via the anaesthetic circuit.

General anaesthesia using muscle relaxant

If the patient is to be intubated, a muscle relaxant is given at the same time as the IV induction agent, or when anaesthesia is reached if the patient has an inhalational induction.

The patient is ventilated via the facemask until the muscle relaxant takes effect. Nitrous oxide and a volatile agent may be added to the gas mix to maintain anaesthesia as the induction agent wears off.

Intubation

The process of introducing an endotracheal tube through the vocal cords into the trachea.

The following are indications for intubation.

- Allow positive pressure ventilation.
- Prevent aspiration: gastric contents, upper airway contaminants (blood, pus).
- Prevent or correct airway obstruction.
- When difficulty is anticipated maintaining the airway by other means (e.g. in patients who are difficult to mask ventilate).
- Ensure a patent airway in operative procedures that provide difficult airway access (prone, head and neck surgeries).
- When operations are performed on the airway itself.

Adverse effects of intubation

- Hypertension, tachycardia, arrhythmia – if anaesthetic too light.
- Damage from the laryngoscope to teeth, lips and tongue.
- Trauma to the larynx or trachea by the tube or cuff – tracheal fistula or stenosis.
- Tube misplacement:
  - Bronchial intubation: the tube is advanced too far and enters a main bronchus thereby ventilating one lung only. Effects include decreased oxygenation, increased CO_2 retention and collapse of the unventilated lung.
  - Oesophageal intubation: the tube is placed in the upper oesophagus rather than the trachea. If not immediately recognised and corrected, hypoxia will result.

Rapid sequence induction (also known as 'crash induction')

Rapid sequence induction ('crash induction') is a modified induction sequence used for patients at risk of regurgitation and aspiration of stomach contents. Unconscious patients and those under general anaesthesia are at risk of aspiration because protective airway reflexes are diminished or lost. Anaesthesia is induced and a fast-onset muscle relaxant is given. Cricoid pressure (posterior pressure on the cricoid cartilage) is applied to compress the oesophagus. The patient is intubated and the endotracheal tube's cuff inflated. This cuff provides protection against soiling of the lower airways.

General anaesthesia without muscle relaxant

Not all operations require the patient to be paralysed for surgical access. General anaesthesia is induced and the patient breathes spontaneously via an anaesthetic facemask or a laryngeal mask airway.

Advantages are the following.

- Faster waking (no need for reversal of neuromuscular blockade).
- No need to intubate – less invasive, lessens associated risks.
- Alerts to light levels of anaesthesia (increased respiratory rate, movement) – less risk of awareness.

Disadvantages are the following.
- No protection against aspiration.
- Patient may have reflex muscle movements and require a deeper plane of anaesthesia for stimulating events.
- CO_2 retention may occur due to decreased respiratory drive under general anaesthesia
- Suitable for:
  - surgeries where muscle relaxation is not required – limb, body surface; and
  - operations lasting less than 3 hours.
- Unsuitable for:
  - those at risk of aspiration;
  - surgery where any patient movement would be disastrous – e.g. neurosurgery;
  - surgery that may produce airway contamination;
  - surgery that restricts access to the airway; and
  - patient positioning that hinders respiratory function and/or respiratory access.

MAINTENANCE OF ANAESTHESIA

During the operation, the patient is continually monitored by the anaesthetist and anaesthetic nurse. Stability of vital signs, depth of anaesthesia, extent of muscle relaxation, fluid balance and maintenance of normal body temperature are all assessed to ensure the patient's safety.

The state of anaesthesia can be **maintained** during the operation in two ways.

- Volatiles: volatile anaesthetic agents are continuously added to the patient's breathing circuit to maintain adequate levels of anaesthesia.

- TIVA (total intravenous anaesthesia): as its name suggests, the patient remains anaesthetised by receiving a continuous IV infusion of anaesthetic agent (Propofol) instead of an inhalational agent.

Muscle relaxants and narcotics are also given as required during the maintenance phase.

PATIENT CARE

Fluid balance

Patients undergoing all but the briefest of procedures will have IV fluid running. Fluid replacement is necessary to counter losses sustained preoperatively (due to fasting or preparations used to cleanse the bowel, which will sustain large fluid loss), and intraoperatively (maintenance fluids and fluid to replace blood loss, fluid loss due to evaporation, and fluid shifts). IV fluids also help keep the cannula patent for drug administration, and help flush and dilute medications. The size of the cannula inserted is influenced by the rate at which fluid needs to be infused. In operations where a large blood loss is expected, a large-bore cannula is used. If blood is to be transfused, a cannula $\geq$ 18g should be inserted.

Types of fluid replacement

- Crystalloids: normal saline, compound sodium lactate (Hartmann's solution), plasmalyte 148 – used for routine fluid replacement.
- Colloids: plasma volume expanders:
  - synthetic: Haemaccel™, Gelinfusin™; and
  - human: plasma protein solution – Albumex 4™.
- Blood products: replace lost blood components.
  - Whole blood: rarely used as usually broken down into component parts:
    packed red blood cells;
    fresh frozen plasma (FFP); and
    coagulation products: platelets, cryoprecipitate, Factor VIII.

Accurate recording of fluid administration is essential. Blood products must be checked to ensure correct patient, blood type, product, product identification number and expiry date.

Urine output

An indwelling catheter is inserted in patients undergoing long procedures, in patients expected to receive large fluid volumes, in patients receiving intraoperative diuretic therapy (e.g. mannitol) or in whom accurate monitoring of urine output is critical (patients with or at risk of renal or cardiac failure, seriously ill patients). Urine is measured and recorded hourly, with the anaesthetist alerted to low volumes (< 60 ml h^{-1}), excessive output (> 200 ml h^{-1}) for adults; and volumes consistent with age and weight for children; or alterations in urine character (blood, concentration, etc.).

Temperature maintenance

Patients undergoing anaesthesia are at risk of developing hypothermia, which can lead to a variety of adverse outcomes. Maintenance of normal body temperature is therefore a priority. The monitoring of central body temperature (as discussed in the 'Monitoring' section) is essential in any case that may put the patient at risk of developing hypothermia.

Mechanisms of perioperative heat loss

- Anaesthetic agents:
  - cause peripheral vasodilation → heat lost from skin;
  - alter the brain's thermoregulatory responses;
  - decrease metabolic rate; and
  - cool, dry gases are administered.
- Muscle relaxants: ↓ muscle movement = ↓ heat production.
- Heat lost to the environment:
  - cool OR;
  - operating table;
  - air currents from air conditioning; and
  - evaporation from the surgical site.
- IV fluids:
  - infusion of cool fluid lowers body temperature; and
  - patients receiving refrigerated blood products are at particular risk.

Maintaining normal body temperature

- Preoperative warming: decreases the initial temperature drop that occurs secondary to the peripheral vasodilation caused by anaesthetic agents.
- Warming IV fluids.
- Insulating the patient: keep the patient covered with blankets.
- Warming irrigation fluids.
- Keep the patient dry: drapes, etc.
- Warm air blowers: transfer heat to the patient.

Pressure area care

Patients undergoing anaesthesia cannot alter their position to relieve pressure on bony prominences, nerves or vessels. A debilitated state preoperatively (malnutrition, weight loss, immobility, impaired vascular function) will increase their risk of pressure area sores, or damage to nerves or vessels from unrelieved pressure. Careful positioning of the patient is essential. Pressure-relieving mattresses should be placed under any patient at risk of developing pressure sores. The ankles may be protected by using padded boots, foam or devices to cradle them off the theatre table. The occiput is protected by a cradling head ring, or by lifting the head off the pillow at regular intervals. Assessment of the patient's skin integrity pre- and postoperatively allows the nurse to plan and evaluate interventions.

MONITORING

Monitoring encompasses the measurement of the patient's physiological variables, the monitoring of the delivery of gases to the patient and the function of the anaesthetic apparatus. It includes both the technical display and the practitioner's vigilance and observation. Continuous monitoring can indicate developing trends and warn of potential problems. However, all monitoring requires skilled interpretation to be of any value.

Visual and auditory alarms on all monitors alert the practitioner to variables outside of the normal range. They can be adjusted to suit individual patient characteristics, but as an important aid to patient safety they should never be turned off.

COMMON PATIENT MONITORS

Oximeter:

- Measures the oxygen saturation of arterial haemoglobin.

Anaesthesia

- Expresses the measurement as a percentage – normal range is 95–100%.

Automated non-invasive blood pressure (NIBP):

- Automatically measures the blood pressure at preset intervals.

Electrocardiograph (ECG):

- Detects electrical activity of the heart and displays it as a waveform.
- Gives the heart rate.
- Shows heart rhythm and allows analysis of arrhythmias.
- Can indicate myocardial ischaemia.

Capnography:

- Measures and displays (numerically, graphically) the inspiratory and expiratory concentrations of CO_2.
- Gas is sampled from the patient's breathing circuit.

The capnography waveform:

- Reflects the phases of ventilation.
- The shape is virtually identical in all healthy patients – an abnormal waveform can be used to determine adverse effects or disease processes.

Other patient monitors

Temperature monitors:

- Anaesthetised patients are at risk of hypothermia – patients being actively warmed are at risk of hyperthermia.
- Continuously monitor and display the patient's core temperature.
- Disposable or reusable thermistor probes are placed in the nasopharynx, oesophagus or rectally; pulmonary artery catheters give core temperature.

Nerve stimulators:

- Measure the neuromuscular blockade by passing an electrical stimulus through a peripheral nerve to evoke a motor response.
- Determine the effect and adequacy of muscle relaxation during anaesthesia.
- Used at emergence to ensure reversal of neuromuscular blockade.

Arterial blood pressure monitor:

- Continuously measures the systemic blood pressure via an intra-arterial cannula.
- Pressure transducer line connected to the cannula sends the information to a monitor.
- Monitor displays the information as a waveform and in numerical form, giving systolic, diastolic and mean arterial pressures.
- Used in cardiac, vascular, neuro, major general surgery; long cases; cases where there may be large blood losses and changes in blood pressure; in patients with cardiovascular disease; in haemodynamically unstable patients; and in patients needing repeated arterial blood gas studies.

Central venous pressure monitor:

- Continuously measures the pressure in the superior vena cava via the central venous catheter and connected pressure transducer line.
- Monitor displays the waveform and numerical central venous pressure reading.
- Reflects right heart filling pressures (preload).
- Gives information on the volume status of the patient.
- Central venous line can also be used for fluid and drug infusions.

Pulmonary artery catheters:

- Balloon-tipped, flow-directed catheter placed via the jugular + subclavian vein, through the superior vena cava, the right atrium and ventricle to the pulmonary artery, where it is wedged. The balloon is then deflated.
- Gives information on central venous pressure, pulmonary artery pressure and pulmonary capillary wedge pressure (which reflects pressure distal to the catheter in the left side of the heart – left ventricle end diastolic pressure).
- Measures cardiac output.
- Gives mixed venous oxygen readings.
- Gives a core temperature reading.
- Highly invasive monitor with many concomitant risks: arrhythmias, cardiac valve injury, pulmonary artery rupture, pulmonary infarction.
- Used in patients with severe cardiac or respiratory disease.

Electroencephalogram (EEG):

- Monitoring of the patient's brain's electrical activity accurately measures the depth of anaesthesia and reduces the risk of awareness.
- Specific anaesthesia EEG monitors use a modified electrode set-up and reflect the level of brain activity as a scale.

Gas analysis:

- Measures and displays in numerical and / or graphical form the inspired and expired concentrations of oxygen, nitrous oxide and anaesthetic volatile agents.
- Gas is sampled from the patient's breathing system.
- Ensures that what is dialled on the anaesthetic machine is what is delivered to the patient.
- Calculates MAC – the minimum alveoli concentration of an anaesthetic vapour (or an anaesthetic vapour plus nitrous oxide) that prevents movement in 50% of the population in response to a standard noxious stimulus. It is used as an index of an anaesthetic agent's potency and allows a comparison between anaesthetic agents.
- Alarms for low inspired oxygen; high anaesthetic agent delivery.

Ventilator monitors:

- Modern ventilators have in-built monitoring systems that measure airway pressures, and an alarm if the pressures are too high or low. Excessive pressure can be caused by inadequate muscle relaxation, poor lung compliance (ARDS, pneumothorax, bronchospasm), too high a tidal volume, or obstruction of the endotracheal tube or circuit. The ventilator also alarms if the airway pressure is below a preset minimum for a set period – this indicates either a circuit disconnection or a large leak in the circuit.

ANAESTHETIC EMERGENCIES

Unexpected adverse events during anaesthesia can occur. Proper recognition and treatment decreases the risk of permanent injury or death. Awareness of potential problems and the steps involved to manage them is essential for the anaesthetic nurse.

AIRWAY

Failure to provide a patent airway can lead to hypoxia, brain and organ damage, and death.

Difficult intubation

The preoperative assessment of the airway will often identify those patients in whom it may be difficult to secure the airway, and alternate plans can be made (awake intubation, gaseous induction, etc.). Every area that provides general anaesthesia should have available equipment to facilitate the difficult intubation. This may be a trolley or basket containing specialised laryngoscope blades, a variety of tubes and laryngeal masks, introducers, equipment for cricothyroidotomy or tracheostomy, and an intubating bronchoscope.

Causes of difficult intubation

To intubate the patient normally, it is necessary to view the vocal cords with the aid of the laryngoscope. The patient is positioned with the neck flexed and the head extended to line up the axis of the pharynx (mouth) and the larynx. The laryngoscope is inserted into the mouth and the tongue is swept to the side. Any anatomical feature that prevents or restricts these movements or alters the anatomy of the upper airway may increase the difficulty of the intubation or render it conventionally impossible.

Some causes are the following.

- Congenital syndromes that alter the anatomy of the face, neck or teeth.
- Anatomical features:
  - short, muscular neck;
  - receding lower jaw;
  - protruding incisors;
  - long, high-arched palate; or
  - shortened distance between the chin and the thyroid cartilage.
- Acquired features:
  - decreased mouth opening: mandibular fractures, dental abscesses, arthritis;
  - restricted neck movement: arthritis, ankylosing spondylitis, cervical spine fractures;
  - soft tissue changes: trauma, burns, tumours, oedema;

Anaesthesia

- obesity; or
- loose teeth in children, missing teeth in adults

Assessment of the airway

Assessment of the patient preoperatively will alert the anaesthetic staff to the presence of any of these features. Perusal of previous anaesthetic records can alert to previous problems.

Further airway assessment

- Mallampati airway classification:[5] the size of the tongue in relation to the oral cavity is visually graded by how much of the pharynx is obscured when the patient sits upright, opens their mouth and protrudes the tongue. There is a correlation between the ability to visualise the pharyngeal structures and the ease of laryngoscopy.
- Neck mobility: the patient is asked to extend and flex the neck.
- Thyromandibular distance: a shortened distance between the chin and the thyroid cartilage is associated with an increased difficulty of intubation.

Despite a thorough preoperative assessment, some patients after induction will present an **unexpected difficult intubation**. Maintenance of patient oxygenation is vital.

Maintain mask ventilation

- Call for help: a more experienced anaesthetist, another anaesthetic nurse to collect difficult intubation equipment.
- Optimise intubation chances: better positioning, different blade or tube, introducer or gum elastic bougie, external laryngeal manipulation.
- Other options
  - awaken the patient (if possible):
  - laryngeal mask airway;
  - continue to mask ventilate for operation;
  - fibreoptic or retrograde intubation; or
  - tracheostomy.
- If the patient is at risk of aspiration, cricoid pressure is maintained until the airway is secured.

Failure to mask ventilate

- Can occur on induction or after multiple intubation attempts. Urgently need to restore oxygen supply to the patient.
- Call for help as above.
- Optimise mask ventilation: 100% O_2, the use of airways, assist in providing good seal around mask, use the emergency oxygen button to provide a high flow oxygen.
- One attempt at intubation should be made.

Or

- Insert the laryngeal mask airway.
- If intubation or the laryngeal mask airway fails to provide a patent airway, perform cricothyroidotomy – an artificial airway inserted through cricothyroid membrane for emergency oxygenation.
- Surgical tracheostomy may now need to be performed to provide a formal airway.
- If at any stage the patient may be wakened to maintain their own airway, this should occur.

Laryngospasm

A reflex partial or complete closure of the vocal cords in the unintubated patient. Occurs secondary to an irritating stimulus during light anaesthesia or during emergence. A 'crowing' noise is heard as air moves past the partially closed cords – in complete spasm, no noise is heard. The patient is difficult or impossible to ventilate. If untreated, oxygen saturation will decrease and the patient will become cyanotic, eventually leading to arrhythmias and cardiac arrest.

Treatment consists of the following.

- 100% oxygen.
- Remove the irritant – suction airway.
- Deepen anaesthesia if too light.
- Positive pressure mask ventilation with a tight-fitting seal.
- If still unable to ventilate – suxamethonium is given to paralyse cords and the patient is intubated.

Bronchospasm

Bronchospasm is a reflex bronchial constriction caused by airway irritants, asthma, anaphylaxis or aspiration. The patient is very difficult to ventilate and a wheeze may be heard. If untreated, oxygen desaturation and cyanosis occurs.

Treatment consists of the following.

- Increase oxygen concentration to maintain adequate oxygenation.
- Remove the stimulus.
- Deepen anaesthesia: volatile agents, though irritating in light anaesthesia, are good bronchodilators.
- Antiasthma drugs: salbutamol (ventolin).
- Adrenaline (for anaphylaxis).

Aspiration

Aspiration is the passage of foreign material into the lungs (especially gastric contents). See 'Rapid sequence induction' for prevention.

Treatment consists of the following.

- Cricoid pressure.
- Suction oropharynx.
- Intubate.
- Suction endotracheal tubes (ETT).
- Chest X-ray to check lung fields.
- Postoperative treatment: may require ICU.

OTHER ANAESTHETIC EMERGENCIES

Scoline apnoea

Scoline (suxamethonium) is a depolarising muscle relaxant. It is broken down by plasma cholinesterase, thereby reversing the muscle blockade. Plasma cholinesterase deficiency, or an alteration in plasma cholinesterase, is a genetically inherited disorder. Patients with altered plasma cholinesterase experience prolonged paralysis after the use of scoline (and mivacurium, a 'newer' non-depolarising short-acting muscle relaxant also broken down by plasma cholinesterase). Treatment is supportive with the patient remaining ventilated until the drug is eventually broken down. Reassurance and sedation are required as the patient, although paralysed, is awake.

Malignant hyperthermia

Malignant hyperthermia is a genetically inherited disorder of skeletal muscle cells that affects the binding of calcium in the sarcoplasmic reticulum. Exposure to trigger agents induces a hypermetabolic state. This may occur on initial exposure to the agent, or after a delay of several hours. Untreated it is often fatal.

Triggers are the following.

- Suxamethonium.
- Volatile anaesthetic agents.
- Amide-type local anaesthetics (lignocaine) have been implicated in the past.

Signs and symptoms are the following.

- Muscle rigidity after injection of suxamethonium (especially masseter spasm – difficulty opening mouth for intubation).
- Increase in end-tidal CO_2.
- Tachycardia, cardiac arrhythmias and cardiac failure.
- Decreased oxygen saturation and cyanosis.
- Metabolic acidosis.
- Electrolyte disturbances: increased potassium and decreased calcium.
- Myoglobinuria: products of muscle breakdown in the urine leading to acute renal failure.
- Rise in temperature: often a late sign, but may increase at $2°C\ h^{-1}$.

Treatment consists of the following.

- Cease all volatile agents.
- Call for assistance.
- Hyperventilate with 100% oxygen via a new anaesthetic circuit (one that has not been exposed to volatile agents).
- Administer Dantrolene to reverse the hypermetabolic process.
- Cool the patient by using cold IV solutions, irrigating the operative site with cold solution and by applying ice packs.
- Correct electrolyte disturbances.
- Administer diuretics and IV fluids to prevent renal failure.

Monitoring consists of the following.

- Arterial line should be inserted to monitor cardiovascular status and to provide access for multiple blood sampling (for acid–base balance, electrolyte testing).
- Temperature probe is inserted.

- Indwelling urinary catheter with an hourly measurement bag is inserted to monitor urine output.
- Follow-up.
  - Patient and members of their immediate family should undergo muscle biopsy to confirm the presence of this genetic disorder.

Cardiac events

The patient's ECG is continually assessed during anaesthesia for heart rate and rhythm. Blood pressure measurements and tissue perfusion are also indicators of effective cardiac function. Adverse cardiac events that can occur during anaesthesia include serious arrhythmias, cardiac ischaemia, myocardial infarction and cardiac arrest. Causes may include the patient's pre-existing cardiac disease, ischaemia secondary to decreased oxygenation (decreased haemoglobin levels, impaired respiratory function), electrolyte disturbances or side-effects from drugs or treatment.

If a cardiac arrest occurs in the operating theatre, call for assistance and the resuscitation ('crash') trolley, which will carry a defibrillator and emergency cardiac drugs. Advanced life-support techniques are followed. The cause of the cardiac arrest, such as electrolyte imbalance or hypovolaemia, is treated simultaneously.

Anaphylaxis

A life-threatening condition resulting from the body's exaggerated immune response to a substance. Can occur following exposure to drugs (induction agents, antibiotics, muscle relaxants), IV contrast dyes, blood or blood products, IV solutions, latex, foods (seafood, peanuts) or stings (bee).

Signs and symptoms are the following.

- Rash, flushing and weals of the skin.
- Oedema of the face and upper airway, progressing to a generalised oedema and fluid shifts.
- Bronchospasm: showing as a wheeze or as difficulty in ventilating.
- Hypotension and tachycardia, progressing to circulatory collapse.

Treatment consists of the following.

- Remove offending stimulus. During anaesthesia, it may be difficult to isolate the offending agent as many drugs are often given in series.
- 100% oxygen.
- Adrenaline in repeated boluses.
- IV fluids.

Follow-up consists of the following.

- Blood samples are taken to confirm the immune response.
- Later testing is conducted to isolate the offending agent.

Awareness

Awareness occurs when the depth of anaesthesia is insufficient. The patient is aware of proceedings, may hear the operating personnel and equipment, and if analgesia is also insufficient, they may feel the pain of surgery. The patient who is muscle paralysed has no means of purposefully responding to this situation. They may become tachycardic and hypertensive. Although a rare occurrence, the psychological trauma experienced by these patients can be overwhelming. Monitors that measure the electrical activity of the brain and assess the depth of anaesthesia are now emerging.

EMERGENCE

At the completion of the operation, the patient needs to be returned to a conscious state. Before transfer out of the operating theatre, the patient must maintain and protect their own airway.

REVERSAL OF NEUROMUSCULAR BLOCKADE

To allow for return of function, the muscle relaxant is ceased before the end of surgery. Any residual blockade is reversed using neostigmine, an anticholinesterase agent. This allows the level of acetylcholine at the neuromuscular junction to build up and a normal impulse transmission to resume. Atropine or glycopyrrolate are given with neostigmine to counter its side-effects (especially bradycardia).

Awakening

IV or volatile agents are turned off. 100% oxygen is given to wash out the nitrous oxide and volatile agent and to provide a respiratory reserve of oxygen for extubation.

Extubation

The patient must be able to maintain their own airway before the artificial airway is removed. The return of normal muscle tone and a rising level of consciousness determines the timing of extubation. Before removal of the endotracheal tube, the oropharynx is suctioned to remove any secretions that may soil the lower airway or irritate the larynx and cause laryngospasm. The patient is placed in the lateral position if there is a risk of vomiting or regurgitation. The air is removed from the cuff of the ETT and the tube is removed. The anaesthetic facemask is applied to provide oxygen and to check the adequacy of the patient's breathing.

Laryngeal mask airway

The IV or volatile agent is discontinued to allow the patient to wake at the completion of surgery. The laryngeal mask airway is removed when the patient obeys commands. The laryngeal mask may be left *in situ* for transfer to the Post-Anaesthetic Care Unit (PACU), and removed there.

Transfer to the PACU

When the patient displays a satisfactory spontaneous respiration and good muscle tone, they may be transferred to their bed or trolley to be taken to the PACU (recovery room).[6] Oxygen therapy is maintained via a clear plastic facemask. Positioning in the lateral position will aid in maintaining a clear airway by allowing the tongue to fall forward and secretions to drain. More awake patients can be positioned according to their comfort. During transport, the patient is monitored visually to ensure regular respiration and the absence of any adverse events.

Once in the PACU, the anaesthetist will outline the type of surgery and anaesthetic, the patient's medical history and postoperative orders to the PACU staff. The anaesthetic nurse should convey any relevant information about the patient's mental status, communication needs, skin integrity or special nursing needs to the PACU nurse taking over his/her care. In the PACU, oxygen therapy is maintained and the patient is assessed for cardio-vascular status, respiratory rate and depth, and level of consciousness. The wound is checked and IV lines, catheters and drains are checked for patency. The patient is assessed for levels of pain or nausea and appropriate interventions are taken.

REGIONAL ANAESTHESIA

Regional anaesthesia is the reversible blocking of nerve conduction, leading to the abolition of sensation. It may be applied to the peripheral nerves or to the spinal cord. Consciousness is retained. Local anaesthetic agents are used that block the sodium channels of the nerve fibres, thereby blocking the impulses passing along them.

COMMON LOCAL ANAESTHETIC AGENTS

Lignocaine:

- Used for spinal, epidural, nerve or plexus blocks, local infiltration, or for topical application.
- Adrenaline can be added to increase the duration of the effect.
- Glucose may be added to produce 'heavy' spinal solutions.
- Rapid onset.
- Moderate duration of effect: 60–90 minutes without adrenaline; 90–120 minutes with adrenaline.

Bupivacaine:

- Used for spinal, epidural, nerve or plexus blocks and local infiltration. Contraindicated in IV regional anaesthesia due to its cardiotoxicity.
- Adrenaline can be added to increase the duration of the effect.
- Glucose may be added to produce 'heavy' spinal solutions.
- Slower onset than lignocaine.
- Long duration of effect (> 3 hours).

Ropivacaine:

- Used in epidural, nerve and plexus blocks and local infiltration.
- Adding adrenaline does not affect the duration.
- Rapid onset.
- Long duration of effect.

Prilocaine:

- Used mainly for IV regional anaesthesia (Bier's Block) due to its relatively low cardiotoxicity. May be used for nerve or plexus blocks or local infiltration.
- 0.5% solution without adrenaline for IV regional anaesthesia.
- Onset and the duration of effect are similar to lignocaine.

Cocaine:

- Used as a topical anaesthetic and vasoconstrictor (nasal mucosa).
- Concentrations of 4–10% solutions.
- Slow onset.
- Duration of effect is 30–60 minutes.

SAFETY TIP: For local infiltration of the digits, penis, ears or nose, solutions containing adrenaline should not be used due to their vasoconstrictor effects.

LOCAL ANAESTHETIC TOXICITY

Local anaesthetic toxicity occurs following IV or intra-arterial injection, or an excessive infiltration dose. Initial symptoms include tongue numbness, perioral tingling, dizziness, slurred speech, tinnitus, restlessness and muscle twitches, progressing to convulsions, unconsciousness and respiratory arrest. Intravascular injection may produce immediate convulsions. Cardiac arrhythmias, profound hypotension and cardiac arrest occur at high systemic levels.

Treatment includes immediate cessation of injection. Patients displaying minor symptoms are watched to check for progression, their cardiovascular status is monitored and oxygen is given. Reassurance and an explanation of symptoms are beneficial. Convulsions are treated with an anticonvulsant (diazepam or thiopentone), and the respiratory and cardiovascular system are supported as needed.

REGIONAL ANAESTHESIA TECHNIQUES

SAFETY TIP: For all regional techniques (other than infiltration of small amounts of local anaesthetics), venous access must be secured before commencement. Resuscitation equipment, including oxygen, a means of ventilating the patient, suction and drugs must be available. The anaesthetic nurse must be aware of potential side-effects and must monitor the patient for these both during the procedure and following its completion.

Topical administration

Used for anaesthesia of the skin or mucous membranes. EMLA™ cream is a lignocaine/prilocaine compound used in paediatrics before IV cannula insertion. Topical lignocaine is applied as a spray, aerosol, gel or ointment for anaesthesia of the skin, nose and airway, and the urethra. Cocaine is used for anaesthesia and vasoconstriction of the nasal cavity.

Infiltration

Local anaesthetics are injected superficially for body surface surgery (e.g. removal of skin lesions), insertion of IV cannulas, dental procedures or to provide postoperative analgesia of the wound site.

IV regional anaesthesia

Used for anaesthesia of a limb (usually upper). Blood is pushed out of the limb using an Eschmarch rubber bandage, and a tourniquet is applied and inflated above arterial pressure. Local anaesthetic (prilocaine) is introduced via an IV cannula already placed in the limb and it produces anaesthesia of the entire limb below the tourniquet. The tourniquet is left inflated during the procedure. Deflation of the cuff within 20 minutes of infiltration can lead to systemic toxicity due to the large amount of local anaesthetic used. Anaesthesia reverses a few minutes after removal of the tourniquet.

A second IV cannula must be placed in a non-operative limb before commencement of anaesthesia.

Nerve blocks

Anaesthesia of the distribution of a nerve can be achieved by injecting local anaesthetic around the nerve proximal to the operative site. Examples include femoral nerve block, digital blocks and retrobulbar (eye) blocks.

Plexus blocks

Infiltrating local anaesthetic in close proximity to a network of nerves will anaesthetise the large area serviced by those nerves. The most commonly performed plexus block is that of the brachial plexus, which gives off many of the principal nerves of the shoulder, chest and arms. The brachial plexus block can be performed at three sites: interscalene (at the interscalene groove on the anterior neck), supraclavicular (above the clavicle) or axillary. The higher the injection site, the greater the extent of the block. Local anaesthesia is distributed around the nerve, causing both a motor and sensory blockade. Because of this total blockade, care must be taken to protect the limb during patient transfer and transport. The block will also provide the patient with immediate postoperative pain relief.

Spinal anaesthesia

Spinal anaesthesia involves the passing of a fine-gauge needle through the dura into the subarachnoid space. A small volume of local anaesthetic agent is injected that comes in contact with the spinal nerves. A complete sensory and motor blockade below that level will result.

The needle is **inserted** below the level of the spinal cord which terminates at L1–2, usually in the third or fourth lumbar space. The needle is inserted under sterile conditions to avoid introducing bacteria to the cerebrospinal fluid (CSF). The patient is positioned either sitting with the back curled or laterally in a fetal position. The curving of the back facilitates needle insertion by opening the intervertebral spaces. The correct position of the needle is ascertained by aspirating CSF. Spread of the local anaesthetic agent can be influenced by patient positioning and by the addition of glucose to the solution to make it 'heavier' than the CSF. Spinal anaesthesia is suitable for operations below the level

of the umbilicus. Since a catheter is generally not inserted, the anaesthetic cannot be 'topped-up'. Therefore, it is appropriate only for operations lasting less than 3 hours. As the patient is awake, spinal anaesthesia is a popular choice for obstetric anaesthesia. It is also a suitable choice for patients unable to tolerate a general anaesthetic due to respiratory disease. It is contraindicated in patients with local or systemic infections due to the risk of CSF contamination. Patients with a fixed cardiac output (aortic stenosis) or hypovolaemia are unsuitable for spinal anaesthesia. Any defect in the patient's coagulation increases the risk of haematoma and cord compression. A pre-existing neurological deficit is a contraindication.

Side-effects are the following.

- Hypotension: occurs due to the concurrent sympathetic blockade, which results in vasodilation below the level of the block. Sudden hypotension may cause the patient to complain of dizziness and nausea. IV fluids are commenced before insertion of the block to preload the vascular compartment. Vasopressors may be given to help maintain the blood pressure. Blood pressure is checked at regular intervals postblock.
- High or total spinal: occurs if an excessive amount of local anaesthetic is injected into the subarachnoid space. The level of the block increases upward, causing widespread paralysis and profound hypotension. If the respiratory muscles are involved, respiratory arrest will occur. If the block is total, the patient will lose consciousness. Treatment includes respiratory support (intubation and ventilation) and treatment of the hypotension (IV fluids and vasopressors).
- Spinal headache: occurs more frequently in younger patients, secondary to leakage of CSF from the dural puncture site. The use of smaller gauge needles diminishes its risk. Treatment involves bed rest (lying flat), adequate fluid intake and simple analgesics. For prolonged severe headache, an epidural blood patch may be performed to seal the leak.
- Urinary retention: may occur after a spinal or epidural anaesthetic. The patient is assessed for postoperative voiding. An inability to void results in the placement of a temporary urinary catheter.

Anaesthesia

Epidural anaesthesia

'Epidural' ('outside the dura') refers to the potential space between the vertebral ligaments and the dura mater of the spinal cord. Spinal nerve roots exit the cord through this space, which also contains veins and some fat. The instillation of local anaesthetic into this space will affect the spinal nerves at the level of injection. Blockade of these spinal nerve roots causes anaesthesia along the length of these nerves (dermatomes). The volume of local anaesthetic injected influences the number and levels of spinal nerves thus affected. The volume and strength of the agent influences the density of the block, with sensory nerves affected first, then motor nerves.

Insertion is done under sterile conditions. The patient is positioned as for a spinal anaesthetic, either sitting or lying laterally. After infiltration of a local anaesthetic into the skin and subcutaneous tissues, a large-bore 'tuohy' needle is inserted and guided between the vertebrae. A special loss of resistance syringe, containing either air or saline, is connected. Continuous pressure is exerted on the plunger of the syringe – as it passes through the ligaments constant resistance is felt. As the needle enters the epidural space, the resistance is lost. A fine catheter is threaded through the needle and left *in situ* in the epidural space. This allows for top-ups of the anaesthetic intraoperatively, and can be left in place for postoperative pain relief.

An epidural anaesthetic may be performed at any level of the spinal column, but is most commonly used for operations below the level of the umbilicus, or for providing postoperative pain relief to the dermatomes of the thoracic or lumbar regions. Epidurals are used to provide analgesia during labour, and are frequently used to provide postoperative pain relief after thoracic or abdominal operations. An infusion is connected to the epidural catheter and a constant rate of local anaesthetic, often with an added narcotic, is given to the patient in the first few postoperative days. The level and density of the block are influenced to provide a sensory-only block to the level of the wound. Patients can mobilise with an epidural infusion, which aids recovery by decreasing the risk of complications associated with prolonged bed rest. Deep breathing and coughing exercises are more readily performed if pain is adequately controlled.

Epidural anaesthesia or analgesia is not appropriate for patients with coagulation defects due to the risk of haematoma formation resulting in cord compression. Infection around the needle insertion site or systemic sepsis is a contraindication. Patients with pre-existing neurological defects may be excluded.

Side-effects are the following.

- Dural puncture: if the tuohy needle is advanced past the epidural space, puncture of the dura may result. Leakage of CSF and headache occur because of the large bore of the tuohy needle. If local anaesthetic is injected a high or total spinal anaesthetic may result (see 'Spinals').
- IV injection: the epidural catheter may be incorrectly placed into an epidural vein. Systemic local anaesthetic toxicity occurs if an anaesthetic agent is injected. Placement of the catheter into an epidural vein may be ascertained by injecting a 'test dose'. A small dose of lignocaine with adrenaline is injected and the patient's pulse rate is monitored. If the catheter is IV, the adrenaline will cause an increase in heart rate. The catheter will then be withdrawn.
- Hypotension: occurs secondary to sympathetic blockade, which causes vasodilation. Treatment is with IV fluids and vasopressors.
- Epidural abscess: occurs rarely. Infection introduced into the epidural space, either during insertion or from migration down the catheter, forms an abscess that compresses the spinal cord. Urgent surgery is required to relieve pressure on the cord and prevent permanent damage.
- Epidural haematoma: occurs rarely. Again, urgent surgery is required to prevent disability.
- Urinary retention: patients may not have a sensation of bladder fullness or may be unable to pass urine. Check for postoperative voiding and the presence of bladder distension. A temporary indwelling catheter may be required.

ANAESTHESIA AND THE ELDERLY PATIENT

As the Western population experiences an ever-increasing life expectancy, a greater proportion of perioperative patients will fall into the category of 'elderly'. Ageing is a normal physiological function that produces changes in the body's appearance, structure and function, and in its ability to adapt to internal and external insults. General consensus marks 65 years as the beginning of old age. However, an individual's chronological age is often not an accurate indicator of their state of health or disease. Although there is a gradual decline in the function of the body's organs from 30 years of age, the environment, lifestyle and genetics will all influence a patient's well being and fitness for anaesthesia and surgery. Each patient must be thoroughly assessed individually, evaluating the reason for the proposed surgery, concurrent medical conditions, medical and surgical history, and current medications. The physical assessment, incorporating the required diagnostic tests (blood tests, ECG, chest X-ray, etc.), monitors the patient for the physiological body system changes associated with ageing.

PHYSIOLOGICAL CHANGES RELATED TO AGEING

Cardiovascular system

The effects of ageing on the cardiovascular system include:

- Decreased cardiac output.
- Loss of compliance of aorta and arterial system.
- Increase in systolic blood pressure.
- Decrease in coronary artery blood flow.
- Decline in maximum heart rate.
- Increased susceptibility to arrhythmias.

Elderly patients with cardiac disease have decreased cardiac reserves and a limited ability to cope with stressors placed on the heart. Coronary artery disease limits the availability of oxygen to the myocardium, leading to ischaemia during times of increased demand. Alterations in peripheral vasculature increase the systolic blood pressure and may lead to left ventricular hypertrophy. Regulation of blood pressure by the elastic nature of the peripheral vessels is lost. The heart's effectiveness as a pump is decreased – circulation time is prolonged and the perfusion of other organs decreases.[7–10]

Anaesthetic considerations

A thorough assessment of the function and limitations of the patient's cardiovascular system will influence the anaesthetic management of the patient. Although each individual's specific needs will dictate the type of anaesthetic, level of monitoring and postoperative management required, anaesthetic care of the elderly will involve the following.

- Preoperative testing: ECG, chest X-ray. Other cardiology tests as required.
- Optimisation of any cardiac conditions preoperatively.
- Continual ECG monitoring intraoperatively.
- IV drugs are given slowly to allow for the patient's prolonged circulation time. Rapid injection of induction agents causes cardiovascular depression and can cause cardiac collapse in the elderly patient with limited compensatory reserve.
- Anaesthetic technique aims to avoid hypotension (decreases perfusion of the myocardium and other organs) and hypertension (increases risk of stroke). Tachycardia is avoided as it increases the oxygen requirements of the heart.
- Supplementary oxygen is continued into the postoperative period to increase availability to the myocardium.[6,7]

Respiratory system and airway management

The effects of ageing on the respiratory system include:

- Rigidity of the chest wall secondary to costal cartilage calcification, kyphosis and osteoporosis.
- Decrease in lung capacities.
- Decreased arterial levels of oxygen.
- Increased susceptibility to infection secondary to decreased immune and ciliary activities.
- Weakening of thoracic muscles decreasing the effectiveness of the cough.[6,7]

Anaesthetic considerations

Assessment of the patient's respiratory function preoperatively will guide the type of anaesthesia given. The elective patient's respiratory status should be optimised before anaesthesia. Medication and chest physiotherapy may be required. The patient must be free of respiratory infections.

8 | Perioperative care of adults

Helen Werder

SURGERY OF THE GASTROINTESTINAL SYSTEM

Abdominal surgery includes surgery of the following.

- Upper gastrointestinal system (oesophagus, stomach, pancreas, small intestine – duodenum, jejunum, ilium, appendix).
- Accessory structures of the hepatobiliary system (liver, gallbladder).
- Spleen.
- Colorectal system (large intestine – caecum, ascending colon, transverse colon, descending colon, sigmoid colon, rectum, anus).
- Structures of the abdominal wall.

These organs are responsible for the process of digestion for the supply of nourishment to the body and for the elimination of solid wastes. Surgery may be performed for exploratory assessment and diagnostic reasons, or to resect a portion of the gastrointestinal system to alleviate obstruction or remove disease.

The **oesophagus** is a muscular tube extending from the pharynx, behind the trachea and heart, through the diaphragm to join the stomach at the cardiac sphincter.

The **stomach** is a dilated section of the alimentary tube situated between the oesophagus and the duodenum, and below the diaphragm. It is divided into three parts – fundus, the body and pylorus – and has two curvatures: the lesser that faces the liver and the greater that faces the abdomen. Attached to the greater curvature is a double fold of peritoneum containing fat called the greater omentum.[1]

The **small intestine** connects to the distal end of the stomach at the pyloric sphincter and continues until it connects to the large intestine at the ileocaecal valve. The proximal section is called the duodenum, which contains a common opening for the common

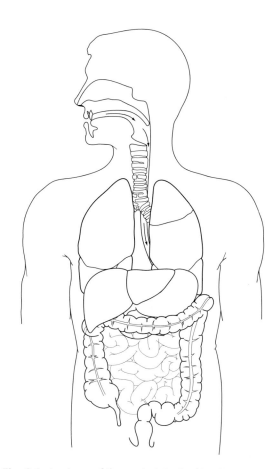

Fig. 8.1 Anatomy of the gastrointestinal tract

bile duct and the pancreatic duct at the ampulla of Vater. The characteristic circular folds of the small intestine mucosa begin in the proximal portion of the duodenum and extend through the jejunum and ilium where they are less prominent. The second section is the jejunum that is situated in the upper abdomen and is continuous with the third section, the ilium, in the lower abdomen. The jejunum and ilium are suspended by the mesentery, which is attached to the posterior abdominal wall. The jejunal circumference is larger and the mucosa is thicker in comparison with the thinner mucosa of the ilium.

The **large intestine** begins in the right iliac fossa at the ileocaecal valve with a small pouch known as the caecum. Attached to the caecum is a blind pouch called the vermiform appendix. Continuous with the caecum is the colon, which is divided into four parts.

- Ascending colon: extends upward from the caecum to the hepatic flexure.
- Transverse colon: lies below the stomach and travels across the abdomen to the splenic flexure.
- Descending colon: extends downwards to just below the iliac crest.
- Sigmoid colon: 'S'-shaped structure that enters the pelvis and terminates in the rectum.

The wall of the colon has three longitudinal strips of muscle distributed around the circumference of the surface with outpouchings of bowel wall between the strips.[1]

The **rectum** extends from the sigmoid colon and ends in the anus. The wall of the rectum consists of four layers similar in structure to the small intestine. The **anal canal** is a narrow passage surrounded and controlled by two circular muscle groups forming the external and internal anal sphincters. The function of the small intestine is the absorption of nutrients whilst the large intestine absorbs water from the contents and expels the solid residue from the body.

The **biliary system** is comprised of the liver, spleen, pancreas and gallbladder. The **liver** lies under the right side of the diaphragm and is divided into the right and left lobes. Located on the inferior surface of the liver is the entry and exit point for the hepatic artery, the hepatic portal vein carrying blood from the digestive system, pancreas and spleen, the common bile duct, and the nerves. The functioning

units of the liver are the more than a million hepatic lobules. Each lobule is supplied by a branch of the hepatic artery and hepatic portal vein, a hepatic duct, nerves and lymphatics, and drained by a central vein. Bile is manufactured in the lobules by the hepatocytes and drains via the tiny bile capillary vessels into the hepatic ducts. These ducts merge to form one common hepatic duct, which then merges with the cystic duct from the gallbladder to form the common bile duct. Bile contains bile salts that facilitate digestion and absorption. The liver functions in the metabolism of carbohydrates, proteins and fats and metabolises nutrients into glycogen stores for regulation of blood glucose levels.[1] The liver also serves in the breakdown of foreign chemicals, and in several important roles in the blood clotting mechanism.

The **gallbladder** is a fibromuscular sac that lies on the undersurface of the right lobe of the liver. The common hepatic duct takes bile to the gallbladder where it becomes highly concentrated during storage. During the digestion of food, the musculature of the gallbladder contracts forcing bile into the cystic duct and through the common duct into the duodenum to aid in digestion by the emulsification of fats.

The **pancreas** lies transversely behind the stomach and is divided into three segments called the head, body and tail. The head is fixed to the curve of the duodenum and shares a common blood supply. The body lies across the vertebrae and extends to the tail, which ends at the hilum of the spleen. The functions of the pancreas are to secrete digestive enzymes via the pancreatic duct into the duodenum, and to secrete hormones (glucagon, insulin) from the cells called the islets of Langerhans into the blood capillaries.

The **spleen** is a large lymphoid organ lying in the left hypochondriac region between the fundus of the stomach and the diaphragm. It is covered with peritoneum that forms supporting ligaments, and is supplied with blood by the splenic artery and drained by the splenic vein into the hepatic portal vein network travelling to the liver. Some of the functions of the spleen are to act as a blood reservoir, to act in defence of the body by phagocytosis of microorganisms, to form non-granular leukocytes and plasma cells, and to act in the phagocytosis of damaged red blood cells.[1]

Perioperative nursing considerations

A preoperative assessment of the patient will enable the OR nurse to assess the patient's history and plan for the operative episode. The assessment will establish that the patient has been informed about the surgical intervention, understands why they need preoperative preparation and understands what is required from them postoperatively. This visit will acquaint the patient with the operative nurse and this information sharing may help to alleviate anxiety and fear of the unknown for the patient.

In planning for the specific needs of the patient, the nurse will identify the following areas for consideration.

- Appropriate positioning of the patient to prevent pressure areas.
- Size of the patient may necessitate extra equipment for safe positioning.
- Additional equipment necessary for safe transferring onto the operating table.
- Size of the patient may necessitate larger and longer instruments and retractors.
- Need for a nurse to remain with the patient until induction is completed to relieve anxiety.
- Need for music in the anaesthetic room to help soothe the anxious patient.
- Extra warming devices may be necessary to prevent hypothermia as large areas of bowel are exposed for lengthy times.
- Fluids needed intraoperatively to be warmed to help prevent hypothermia.
- Jelly-filled mattresses needed to prevent pressure areas.
- Recording of all intraoperative fluid losses to prevent fluid volume deficits.
- Maintenance of an aseptic technique to reduce the risk of infection.
- Appropriate containment of contaminants.
- Keeping the room temperature at a level that provides for maintenance of body temperature.
- Need for removal of hair from the incision site as close as possible to the commencement of the operation.
- Need for an indwelling catheter to be inserted after induction.
- Safe site for application of the diathermy plate.

SURGICAL INTERVENTIONS

Surgical procedures involving the structures of the gastrointestinal system usually involve an abdominal incision, but many procedures are performed using endoscopic and laparoscopic interventions. The decision about which approach to choose to enter the abdominal cavity is dependent on what may afford maximum exposure of the involved structures and provide minimal postoperative pain and discomfort to the patient. The surgical technique involved in opening and closing abdominal incisions is reflected in successful achievement of this result.

Some of the common surgical interventions for gastrointestinal surgery are the following.

- Laparotomy or laparoscopy for diagnostic reasons, which may proceed to further operative procedures to resect or remove diseased organs.
- Open cholecystectomy or an appendicectomy to resect or remove organs.
- Repair of a hernia, which is a reparative procedure.

Types of abdominal incisions

The **vertical midline incision** either above the umbilicus, below the umbilicus or full length around the umbilicus is the most common preferred incision because it offers good exposure to most structures in the abdominal cavity. It transverses the fewest layers and can be closed joining the peritoneum and posterior fascia as a single layer, and the anterior fascia, subcutaneous tissue and skin as individual layers.

The **McBurney incision** involves a small oblique incision that begins well below the umbilicus, goes through McBurney's point, and extends upward toward the right flank. It is most commonly used for removal of the appendix. The access provided does not allow good exposure and involves splitting of the external, internal and transversalis muscles and fascias in the direction of their fibres. It is easy and quick to close and provides a firm wound closure.[1]

The **subcostal incision** is usually made on the right side for operations on the gall bladder, common duct or pancreas and on the left side for a splenectomy. Unless extended, it only gives limited exposure but has the advantages of giving less tension of the incision edges and less respiratory impairment.[1]

The **Pfannenstiel incision** involves a slightly curved incision just above the symphysis pubis and is used for pelvic surgery.

The **mid-abdominal transverse incision** can be either right or left sided and is used for a retroperitoneal approach. It can start either above or below the umbilicus and is angled between the ribs and iliac crest to the lumbar region. The muscles are both divided and split but have good alignment when the rectus sheath is sutured.

The **thoracoabdominal incision** is used to gain access to the proximal portion of the stomach and the distal section of the oesophagus. After the patient is positioned on the unaffected side, the incision starts from a point midway between xiphoid process and umbilicus and extends across the costal margin and along the eighth intercostal space. Both the costal cartilage and the diaphragm are divided to expose the stomach.

The **bilateral upper abdominal transverse incision** is an inverted 'U' in shape and extends from a point below the costal margin in line with the anterior axillary line on one side to a similar point on the opposite side. It is used for biliary and pancreatic procedures and especially for liver transplantation where wide exposure is required to both the liver and upper gastrointestinal regions.

The **inguinal incision** is either a right or left oblique incision in the inguinal region giving exposure of the structures in the groin region. The muscles involved are the external and internal obliques, the transversus abdominis, the conjoined tendon, and the external inguinal ring.[2]

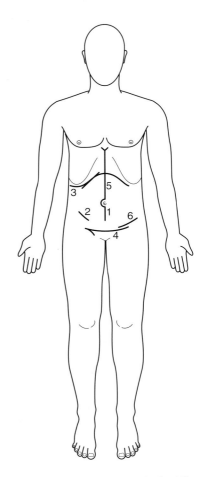

Fig. 8.2 Abdominal incisions: 1, vertical midline; 2, McBurney; 3, subcostal; 4, Pfannenstiel; 5, bilateral upper abdominal transverse; 6, inguinal

Laparotomy

A laparotomy is the surgical incision through the abdominal wall to gain access to the contents of the peritoneal cavity for gastrointestinal surgery. Surgical intervention may be indicated for diagnostic, therapeutic, palliative or prophylactic reasons. The procedure may be necessary to repair or remove traumatised tissue, to cure disease processes by organ and tissue removal, and/or to examine by biopsy or otherwise internal organs for diagnosis.[1]

The patient is placed in a supine position with one or both arms supported on armboards. The skin is prepared from the nipple line to the upper third of the thighs and to the bedline laterally with antimicrobial solution. A vertical midline incision is made through the skin to the fascia using a scalpel. Haemostasis is obtained using electrocoagulation, ligating clips or absorbable ligatures. The fascia is incised and the external oblique muscle split and retracted. After haemostasis is controlled, the internal oblique and transverse muscles are split parallel to the fibres and up to the rectus sheath. The peritoneum is grabbed with plain forceps, a nick made with a knife, and then the incision is extended with scissors up and down the full length of the wound. After a brief exploration of the abdominal contents is made, a self-retaining retractor is then inserted over the wound edges to maintain adequate exposure. This is the initial step in gastrointestinal surgery with following procedures dependent on the type of surgery to be performed.

Resection of a tumour or the removal of an organ has traditionally been carried out using suture materials such as chromic, silk, synthetic absorbable and non-absorbable suture material. Surgical stapling instruments have greatly impacted on the technical aspects of gastrointestinal surgery. This technology has replaced conventional suturing techniques to a great extent. The stapling instruments can be employed to divide and ligate, resect and anastomose with the design of the implanted staple not compromising the vascularity of the resected tissue edges.[1] These devices are available in reusable and disposable models. Operative nurses must be familiar with the assembly and loading of this equipment.

The anastomosis used for rejoining bowel is dependent on achieving the best outcome with the available gastrointestinal tract remaining. The anastomosis used may be a direct end-to-end joining of the bowel as used for a hemicolectomy, an end-to-side joining as in the remaining stomach being attached onto the jejunum after a partial gastrectomy, or a side-to-side anastomosis between the ileum and transverse colon after a hemicolectomy. Regardless of which anastomosis is chosen, the purpose is to form a continuous conduit for the processing of food from the mouth to the anus.

To close the laparotomy, tissue forceps (Littlewood's) or clamps are placed along the peritoneal tissue edges to approximate the edges. The peritoneum is closed with a continuous or interrupted absorbable suture. The muscle tissue is approximated and may or may not be sutured. The external oblique fascia is closed with interrupted sutures and the subcutaneous layer may or may not be sutured. The skin edges are approximated with tissue forceps and sutured with a non-absorbable suture such as nylon or joined with skin staples.

A permanent or temporary outlet for the gastrointestinal tract may be required after some types of surgery. This outlet (either a colostomy or an ileostomy) may be for resting the bowel or as a replacement for the functions of the anus. This outlet is achieved by bringing part of the small or large intestine to the surface via an opening on the abdominal wall and suturing the stoma in place. Similarly, an alternative method of gaining nutrition (gastrostomy) may be required when the alimentary tract from the mouth to the stomach needs to be rested or remain unused for a period. This is achieved by placing a gastrostomy feeding tube from the skin of the abdominal wall into the gastric lumen. This may be a temporary, permanent or palliative procedure to prevent malnutrition or starvation.

Surgery for diseases of the liver, biliary tract, pancreas and spleen that attach to the gastrointestinal tract may be performed for tumours, infection, congenital anomalies, cystic anomalies, metabolic diseases or trauma. Resection of carcinomas of the liver has a high success rate for cure and new technology has enabled successful organ transplantation for the liver, pancreas and kidneys.

Laparoscopic intervention

Cholecystectomy is a commonly performed operation in most operating rooms for removal of gallstones. Laparoscopic cholecystectomy has become a popular method of surgical intervention for the treatment of cholecystitis. Following the success of this operation, there has evolved a large number of abdominal procedures now being performed or assisted through the laparoscope. The advantages of laparoscopic intervention are the reduction of postoperative ileus, and a shortening of the recovery period and hospitalisation.

Perioperative nursing considerations for laparoscopic surgery

The preoperative evaluation for laparoscopic patients varies little from that of a patient scheduled for a laparotomy and the same points should be considered. The patient is positioned in a supine position but may be tilted into a reverse Trendelenburg position intraoperatively. Other aspects for consideration during these procedures are the following.

- Laparoscopic procedure may convert to a laparotomy at any time and the appropriate instrumentation should be available.

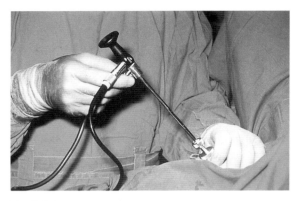

Fig. 8.3 Laparoscopy

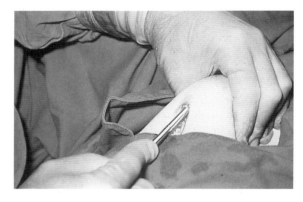

Fig. 8.4 Laparoscopy

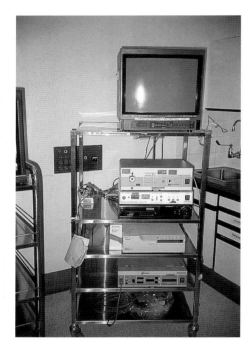

Fig. 8.5 Laparoscopic tower

- Patient must be made aware of this possibility.
- Laparoscopic instrumentation and equipment should be assembled and be in good working order before commencement.
- Laparoscopic camera, camera unit, insufflator, monitor, light source and video unit should be tested before commencement.
- Insufflation pressure must be set to 15 mmHg as exceeding this may lead to changes in blood pressure, bradycardia or the development of gas emboli in an exposed blood vessel.
- Pressure flow of the CO_2 gas should not exceed $2\,l\,min^{-1}$.
- Suction and electrosurgical equipment should be in good working order.
- A method for defogging the laparoscope should be available, e.g. warm water.

Laparoscopic intervention

The basic laparoscopy involves the making of a small incision in the fold of the umbilicus through which a percutaneous needle or trocar and sheath are placed. The peritoneal cavity is insufflated with warmed CO_2 and a rigid wide-angle laparoscope is placed into the operative sheath for direct visualisation of the abdominal viscera.[1] This initial visualisation can be for diagnostic purposes or as part of the surgical intervention when additional operative ports are introduced to facilitate the introduction of operative instrumentation and suction. The placement of these additional ports will depend on the locality of the organ that is to be operated on. Laparoscopic procedures are commonly performed for cholecystectomy, appendicectomy, herniorrhaphy, nissenfundoplication, bowel resections, laparoscopically assisted oesophagectomy and tubal ligations.

Open cholecystectomy

An open cholecystectomy is the removal of the gall-bladder. This surgical procedure is performed for

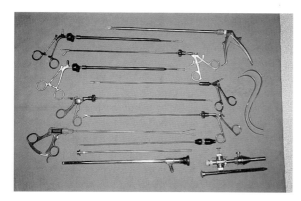

Fig. 8.6 Laparoscopic instruments

acute or chronic cholecystitis, cholelithiasis or to treat carcinoma. The common duct is left intact so that a functional pathway is available for the elimination of bile via the duodenum. An intraoperative cholangiogram will usually be performed during this procedure. Therefore, an operating table prepared to take X-rays and X-ray gowns or lead shields must be used. The cholangiocath, equipment and contrast medium for the procedure should be available and the surgical team should ensure the patient has not had any allergic reactions to the contrast medium on previous occasions.

The patient is placed in a supine position with the arms extended on armboards. The skin is prepared with an antimicrobial solution from the nipple line superiorly to the iliac crest inferiorly, and from the bedline on the right side to the nipple line on the opposite side. Through a right subcostal incision, the abdominal cavity is opened. Haemostasis is obtained with electrosurgical coagulation, then a moist sponge is placed over the liver and the liver is retracted gently upwards with a broad Deaver retractor. The pathology is determined and if the gallbladder is greatly distended, it may be drained by inserting a trocar attached to suction. The stab wound will be clamped to prevent leaking of bile and the instrument will be isolated in a dish. The gallbladder is grasped in a forceps for gentle traction and manipulation. The cystic duct, common bile duct, and hepatic artery and any branches are identified and dissected from surrounding structures using blunt and sharp dissection. Haemostasis is maintained with electrosurgical coagulation. The hepatic artery

and any branches are doubly clamped and ligated with non-absorbable suture material or ligating clips.

At this stage, an intraoperative cholangiogram may be performed to assess patency of the common bile duct and to identify stones in the hepatic and common bile ducts. The cholangiocath is prepared by flushing the catheter and tubing with normal saline to eliminate air bubbles. A small incision is made into the cystic duct and the catheter inserted and anchored in the common bile duct by the surgeon's preferred method. Flushing during insertion facilitates dilatation of the duct. The syringe of normal saline is exchanged for a syringe containing contrast medium diluted with normal saline. When the surgeon is ready to perform the X-ray, sponges and instruments that might interfere with visualisation of the contrast medium are removed and the operative site is covered with a sterile drape. The X-ray equipment is positioned and the surgeon will direct the radiology technician about when to take the radiograph. After the radiograph has been taken, the drape is removed in a manner so as not to contaminate the sterile field or the nurse. The X-ray is viewed immediately it has been developed and a decision made about whether the operation will proceed, if more X-rays are required or if to explore the common bile duct.

The moist sponge packs and retractors are reinserted and the operation proceeds. The cystic duct is doubly clamped, ligated and divided. The gallbladder

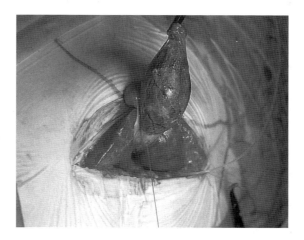

Fig. 8.7 Cholecystectomy

is freed from the liver bed working upward towards the fundus and removed. Haemostasis is achieved using electrosurgical coagulation. A closed suction drain is inserted and exteriorised through a stab wound in the abdominal wall and the wound closed in layers. Dressings are applied to the wound and the drain site. This operation may also be performed laparoscopically.

Appendicectomy

An appendicectomy is the removal of the appendix. The procedure is performed to remove an acutely inflamed appendix and therefore to prevent peritonitis.

The patient is placed in the supine position with one or both arms supported on armboards. The skin is prepared with antimicrobial solution as for a laparotomy. A right lower quadrant incision (McBurney) is made and the muscles retracted with Langenbeck retractors. The peritoneum is grasped with artery forceps and a small incision made with a knife and extended with scissors. Free fluid within the peritoneal cavity is swabbed and sent for culture and sensitivity testing. The appendix is identified and grasped with a Babcock forceps for gentle traction. Sponges may be placed around the base of the appendix to avoid contamination of the remaining bowel if rupture occurs. The mesoappendix is dissected from along the appendix by separating and clamping small sections of tissue and ligating with absorbable ties. The base of the appendix is grasped with a Babcock forceps and a straight Harrison Cripp clamped across the base crushing the stump. The appendix is excised and removed and the stump

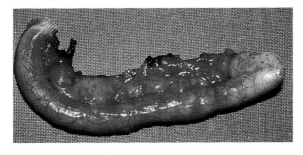

Fig. 8.8 Appendicectomy: an inflamed appendix

ligated. The stump may be inverted into the caecum by placing a purse-string suture around the base and pulling it closed, or the stump may be cauterised with electrosurgical coagulation, or swabbed with an antimicrobial solution or the stump may be left alone. The appendix, instruments and swabs used during the amputation are placed immediately into a kidney dish and passed from the sterile field. The peritoneal cavity is irrigated with a large amount of warm normal saline. The wound is closed in layers and the appendix sent as a specimen to pathology. Appendicectomies may also be performed laparoscopically.

Hernia repair

A herniorrhaphy is the repair of a herniation of the abdominal contents caused by a musculofascial defect in the abdominal wall or groin area.[2] A hernia can involve protrusion of a portion of the parietal peritoneum but often includes a part of the intestine. The most frequent places of occurrence are the inguinal canals, the femoral rings and the umbilicus. Hernias can be congenital defects or have other contributing factors to their formation such as age, sex, previous surgery, nutritional state, obesity, and pulmonary and cardiac disease.[1] Hernias can be classified as reducible where the contents of the sac can be returned to the normal intra-abdominal position or irreducible (incarcerated) where the contents of the sac are trapped outside the abdomen and may become strangulated. In the inguinal/femoral region, direct and indirect hernias are two types of herniation that commonly occur. A direct hernia is where the peritoneum bulges through the fascia in the groin area and the sac may contain abdominal viscera. An indirect hernia is more likely to be caused by a congenital defect in the internal abdominal ring, causing the peritoneum to bulge along the spermatic cord. It may or may not contain abdominal viscera.

For an inguinal hernia, the patient is placed in a supine position with one or both arms supported on armboards. The skin is prepared with an antimicrobial solution as for a laparotomy. A left or right oblique incision is made in the groin area and dissection continued with scissors until the hernia is exposed. In the male, the fascia overlying the spermatic cord is incised and the edges of the fascia

development of secondary sexual characteristics. The corpus luteum secretes the hormone progesterone that is essential for the implantation of the fertilised ovum and the development of the embryo.[1]

The vagina is a collapsed tube lined with mucous membrane extending from the cervix to the external surface of the body. The entrance to the vagina is partially or fully covered by folds of mucosa called the hymen. The vagina has the bladder and ureters in close proximity anteriorly, and the rectum posteriorly. It functions as the excretory duct for products of menstruation, as the birth canal and as the organ for copulation.

Oestrogen produced during puberty deposits fatty tissue over the symphysis pubis. This mound called the mons pubis also becomes covered with hair at this time. Extending downward and backward from the mons pubis to the perineum are two folds of skin called the labia majora with hair on their outer surface and a smooth inner surface moistened by large sebaceous glands. The labia minora comprise two folds of hairless skin that lie within the labia majora. Anteriorly, the labia minora form the prepuce of the clitoris laterally, and the frenulum medially. The clitoris is the homologue of the penis in the male[1] but does not contain the urethra. The labia minora surround a smooth area called the vestibule that contains the openings for the urethra and the vagina. The urethral opening is called the urethral meatus and lying on either side of this are two of the vestibular glands called the Skene's glands. Another two vestibular glands called the Bartholin's glands are on either side of the vaginal orifice with the ducts opening into the inner aspects of the labia minora. The vestibular glands because of their location are subject to infections.

The perineum is a skin-covered muscular area between the vaginal opening and the anus. During childbirth, this region can be torn and weaken the support system of the vaginal area resulting in partial vaginal or uterine prolapse.[2]

Surgery on any of these reproductive organs is performed for diagnostic purposes in instances of abnormal bleeding from these organs, for suspected malignant or benign tumours and for infertility. Surgery can also be performed for therapeutic purposes when repairs are required to strengthen weakened structures or to remove others.

Perioperative nursing considerations

The nursing assessment for patients undergoing gynaecological surgery should involve the routine questions but particular attention should be paid to consent especially when organs are to be removed. Attention should also be paid to cultural and religious beliefs and these should be incorporated into the nursing plan for maintenance of privacy during the operative phase. Consideration should also be given to the psychological issue of body image. Many women may experience feelings of loss of self-worth when their organs of reproduction are removed. The perioperative nurse should identify the patient's strengths, give information relevant to her perceived body image alterations, and offer empathy and positive regard.[1]

Other nursing interventions may include the following.

- An assessment of the size of the patient may identify a need for longer surgical instruments.
- Ensuring any results from tests and scans ordered are present in the operating theatre (e.g. MRI or CAT scans that identify the extent of suspected malignancy).
- Identify the mobility of the patient's joints and the condition of the skin if the patient is to be placed in a lithotomy position.
- Ensure the appropriate positioning aids are available.
- Identify the need for a urinary catheter.
- Ensuring a warming mattress is available as some procedures can be lengthy and the opening of the abdominal cavity will increase the loss of heat from the body.
- Selection of an appropriate electrosurgical dispersive pad site.

SURGICAL INTERVENTION

Gynaecological surgery may be performed with either the abdominal or vaginal approach or by an abdominovaginal approach. The most common surgical procedures in gynaecology are the D&C (dilatation and curettage), vaginal anterior and posterior repair, vaginal hysterectomy, laparoscopy with or without tubal ligation, and the abdominal hysterectomy.

Vaginal procedures

Operations for vaginal procedures are usually performed with the patient in a lithotomy position with the surgeon either standing or seated. The bladder may or may not be drained before the procedure and an indwelling catheter may or may not be left *in situ* after the procedure. Care should be taken that the sacral area is padded to prevent pressure areas developing. The legs should be slowly raised and lowered together to prevent disturbances caused by rapid alterations in venous return and injury to the rotator hip joint.[2]

Dilatation and curettage (D&C)

This procedure is the gradual enlargement of the cervical os and the curetting of endometrial or endocervical tissue for histological study. It may be performed to control dysfunctional bleeding or to complete an incomplete abortion, or for diagnosing cervical or uterine malignancy, or for investigating infertility. Multiple specimen containers should be available for specimens. A D&C instrument set will be necessary and a gynaecological table as well as the instrument table.

The area should be prepared with an antimicrobial solution from the mons pubis backward towards the anus and laterally to mid-thigh. A Sims speculum may be placed anteriorly and retracted to expose the cervix. The anterior lip of the cervix is grasped with a tenaculum / vulsellum forceps and a graduated sound is passed through the uterine canal into the cavity to determine its depth and direction. Using Hegar dilators, the surgeon will dilate the cervical canal

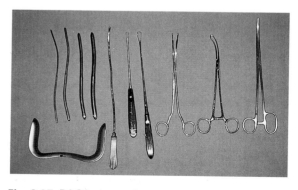

Fig. 8.17 D&C instruments

increasing in size each dilator. A curette is used gently to scrape the uterine cavity either partially or more fully. The curettings are collected on a gauze square on the weighted speculum. If a cervical malignancy is suspected, then the endocervical curettings are taken before uterine curettings. When the uterus is evacuated after an incomplete abortion, a curved sponge holder or large blunt curette may be introduced to remove remaining tissue. The tenaculum / vulsellum and retractors are removed, the patient is cleaned and dressed with a perineal pad.

Anterior and posterior repair

A reconstructive repair of the vagina is performed to correct a cystocele, enterocele or a rectocele and to restabilise the support of the anterior and posterior vaginal walls. Obstetric trauma, age or an inherent weakness[1] may cause these defects. Vaginal instrumentation and a D&C set will be required. The patient should be prepared with an antimicrobial solution from the lower abdomen above the mons pubis anteriorly to the anus posteriorly, and to mid-thigh laterally.

The internal vaginal structures are exposed using vaginal retractors. The tissue between the bladder and vagina at the bladder reflection is exposed and the full thickness of the vaginal wall is separated up to the bladder neck. The edges of the cystocele are grasped with Allis forceps and retracted away from the operative area. The urethra and bladder neck are mobilised and if repairs are necessary to the bladder neck, urethra or cervix, they are carried out at this stage. The edges of the cystocele are trimmed of excess stretched tissue and the anterior vaginal wall is sutured closed.

Tissue forceps are placed posteriorly on either side at the mucocutaneous junction and skin and mucosa are excised and dissected from the muscles beneath. Another tissue forceps is placed centrally on the posterior vaginal wall and retracted to permit further dissection from the posterior vaginal fornix. The perineum is dissected from attached tissue posteriorly. The rectocele is reduced and the posterior vaginal wall is trimmed of excess tissue. The rectocele is repaired and the muscles sutured to strengthen the repair. The trimmed mucosal edges are sutured with interrupted sutures and a vaginal pack and indwelling catheter may be inserted.

Vaginal hysterectomy

A vaginal hysterectomy is the removal of the uterus via a vaginal approach. This procedure is performed when there is a benign tumour and the uterus is not enlarged. It would be contraindicated if a malignancy involving the fallopian tubes or ovaries were involved and when the extent of the disease is not known. The patient will be positioned in a lithotomy position with a slight Trendelenburg. The skin preparation will be as for an anterior and posterior repair.

A retractor is placed in the vagina and the labia may be retracted to facilitate vision of the interior of the vagina. A suture or clamp (vulsellum or tenaculum) is placed on the lip of cervix to permit traction. A circular incision is made around the cervix in the vaginal tissue. The bladder is dissected off the anterior surface of the cervix and the peritoneum of the anterior and posterior cul-de-sacs is incised. The uterosacral ligament and blood vessels are clamped, ligated and cut. Whilst retracting the bladder aside, the cardinal ligament and uterine arteries are double clamped, ligated and cut and the uterus is delivered. Preserving the ovarian vessels, the remaining structures in the broad ligaments on either side are clamped and cut and the entire specimen is removed, then the pedicle is ligated. Repairs to any structures are carried out at this stage and the peritoneum is closed using an absorbable suture. An indwelling catheter may be inserted and the vagina may be packed.

Laparoscopy

A laparoscopy is the insertion of an endoscope through the anterior abdominal wall to visualise the peritoneal cavity following the establishment of a pneumoperitoneum. Laparoscopy is usually performed for diagnostic investigation of pelvic pain, for investigating infertility, for evaluating pelvic masses, or identifying ectopic masses, and for elective sterilisation procedures.

The patient will be positioned in a lithotomy position and the abdomen, perineum and vagina will be prepared with an antimicrobial solution and draped. Instrumentation for a laparoscopy and a D&C should be prepared and a laparotomy set available. The bladder may be emptied before commencing and a dilatation and curettage may be performed at this stage.

After sounding the depth and direction of the cervix a Spachmann cannula is introduced into the cervix either to manipulate the uterus for better visualisation or for the introduction of a dye during infertility diagnostic procedures. A small incision is made in the inferior margin of the umbilicus. The skin may be elevated by the placement of tissue grasping forceps on either side of the umbilicus and retraction or by the surgeon grasping below the umbilicus and applying lifting traction. A Verres needle is passed through the incision into the peritoneal cavity and after confirming correct placement a pneumoperitoneum is established with approximately two litres of carbon dioxide gas. Correct placement is confirmed by connecting a partially filled syringe of saline and aspirating. After withdrawing the Verres needle a trocar and sleeve is introduced downward towards the pelvis, the trocar is withdrawn and the carbon dioxide gas tubing is reconnected to maintain the pneumoperitoneum.

A laparoscope is introduced into the sleeve and the light cable connected. The contents of the peritoneal cavity can now be visualised. If a laparoscopic assisted sterilisation is to be performed, a second centimetre incision is made suprapubically for additional instruments to be introduced into the cavity. If the fallopian tubes are being tested for patency, then methylene blue diluted in 20 ml saline is introduced via the Spachmann cannula and the exit observed through the fimbriated ends. After completion of the procedure, the laparoscope is removed and gas is allowed to escape via the trocar. A subcuticular stitch is placed in the incisions and the wounds covered with a Steri-strip or Band-aid. The Spachmann cannula is removed and a perineal pad placed *in situ*.

Abdominal hysterectomy

An abdominal hysterectomy is the removal of the entire uterus through an abdominal incision. At this time removal of the ovaries and fallopian tubes may also be performed (salpingo-oophorectomy). A hysterectomy may be performed for endometriosis, pelvic inflammatory disease, dysfunctional bleeding, postmenopausal bleeding, fibroids, malignant tumours, and for sterilisation.

The patient's position is supine or Trendelenburg with arms extended on armboards. The vagina may

Perioperative care of adults

be prepared and the bladder may be emptied; therefore instruments should be available for this procedure. The patient is prepared with an antimicrobial solution from the umbilicus to the upper thigh and laterally to the bedline. The operation can be performed through a midline or paramedian incision, but is mostly performed through a lower transverse or Pfannenstiel incision.

The procedure to gain entrance into the peritoneal cavity is the same as for a laparotomy. After the peritoneum is opened, the wound edges will be covered with sponges and a self-retaining retractor inserted. The bowel will be packed away upwards with large warm moist sponges and the patient positioned in a slight Trendelenburg. It should be noted that heavy gynaecological clamps such as Heaney, Kocher and Harrison Cripps will be used and cutting will be with a knife or heavy Mayo scissors. Suture material will be absorbable and an individual suture will be used each time with the length of suture material often left attached for traction. Care should be taken not to remove clamps too quickly as large vessels are being ligated and haemorrhage will result if the ligating material has not been tightened.

The round ligaments are clamped, ligated and cut with the suture material left long for traction. The layer of the broad ligament close to the uterus is separated with the surgeon's fingers and haemostasis maintained. Clamping the utero-ovarian ligaments and the fallopian tubes together, the surgeon will incise and double ligate the tissue to isolate the uterus. The posterior sheath of the broad ligament is exposed, the ureters are identified, and then the uterine vessels and uterosacral ligaments are double-clamped, incised and ligated. The uterus is mobilised to the level of the bladder, then the bladder is separated from the cervix and upper vagina by dissecting the peritoneal covering away from the bladder.

At the level of the cervix, the cervix is clamped with Kocher clamps or grasped with Allis forceps. The uterus is dissected from the vaginal vault using scissors or a knife. The uterus is removed together with any potentially contaminated instruments from the sterile field. If the uterus is to be removed by the use of a stapling device, the vaginal vault is left closed to prevent contamination of the peritoneal cavity.

If surgical staples have not been used, closure of the vagina is achieved with several layers of an absorbable suture. The bladder is reperitonealised and the peritoneum is closed over the vaginal vault and rectum. After irrigating the peritoneal cavity with warm saline, the omentum and bowel are returned to their anatomical position. A drain may be inserted and the abdominal wound is closed as for a laparotomy.

SURGERY OF THE GENITOURINARY SYSTEM

Genitourinary surgery involves procedures of the male and female urinary system, and because of its close anatomical association, procedures of the male reproductive system. The urinary organs consist of a pair of kidneys, two ureters, the urinary bladder and the urethra. The male reproductive organs consist of the scrotum that contains the paired testes and epididymis; the vas deferens, the seminal vesicles, ejaculatory ducts, the bulbourethral glands, the prostate gland, penis and the urethra (common to both systems).

The kidneys are situated in a retroperitoneal location on the posterior wall of the abdominal cavity, one on each side of the vertebral column. The right kidney is slightly lower than the left because of the liver situated above it. The kidney has three

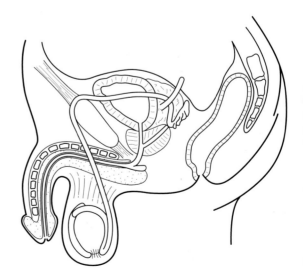

Fig. 8.18 Anatomy of the male genitourinary and reproductive system

regions, the cortex, the medulla and the pelvis. The renal artery and renal vein enter and leave the kidney on the medial side at a concave area called the hilum. On entering the kidney the renal artery divides many times until they become small afferent branches which pass to the glomeruli. Efferent arterioles in the glomeruli then pass to the tubules of the nephron.[1] The tubules funnel urine into the calyces that channel urine into the renal pelvis. Each kidney is capped on the superior medial surface with an adrenal gland. The medulla of the gland secretes adrenalin, and the cortex secretes steroids and hormones.

The ureters transport urine from the renal pelvis of the kidney to the urinary bladder. The ureters leave the renal pelvis and descend between the parietal peritoneum and the body wall to the pelvic cavity. Here they turn medially and enter the urinary bladder on its posterior lateral surface.[2] The middle muscular layer of the ureters has an inner mucosal layer and an outer fibrous layer. An accumulation and distension by urine of this muscular layer initiates a peristaltic action that propels urine down the ureter into the urinary bladder.

The urinary bladder is a hollow muscular organ that acts as a reservoir for urine. It is retroperitoneal and is situated behind the pubic symphysis and anterior to the rectum in males and to the uterus and upper vagina in females. The ureters enter the bladder at a smooth muscular region called the trigone of the bladder with the urethral orifice making up the third corner of the triangle. The bladder has three layers of smooth muscle and is lined with transitional epithelium. Micturition occurs when distension of the bladder initiates a response from the autonomic nervous system which results in contraction of the bladder muscles and relaxation of the bladder outlet sphincters.

The urethra extends from the inferior surface of the urinary bladder and exits at the tip of the penis in males and to the external urinary meatus located between the clitoris and the vaginal orifice in females. It is a muscular tube lined with mucous membrane, approximately 4 cm long in females and 20 cm in males. The male urethra has three distinct parts, the prostatic, membranous, and spongy sections which are named according to the regions through which it passes. The bulbourethral glands (Cowper's glands) enter the spongy urethra a short distance below the urogenital diaphragm or pelvic floor.[2]

The scrotum is a skin covered muscular pouch that holds the oval-shaped organs of sperm production called the testes. Besides producing spermatozoa, specialised cells called Leydig cells produce the male hormone testosterone. Each testis consists of many tubules that condense in number and continue into the adjacent epididymis where the sperm mature and are stored.[1] The epididymis is a convoluted duct located along the posterolateral surface of the testis. It has smooth muscles in the wall that contract during ejaculation and it secretes seminal fluid which provides a liquid medium to aid the sperm in their migration. The vas deferens is the distal continuation of the epididymis and it forms the spermatic cord as it joins the testicular vessels and nerves on entering the abdominopelvic cavity. The vas deferens is joined by a duct of the seminal vesicles to form the ejaculatory duct which then passes through the prostate gland and opens into the posterior urethra. The seminal vesicles produce protein and fructose to nourish the sperm cell. At the time of ejaculation, sperm and prostatic fluid are both ejaculated.

The prostate gland is a fibromuscular organ that encompasses the urethra just below the bladder and anterior to the rectum. The lobes of the prostate gland secrete highly alkaline fluid that dilutes the testicular secretion as it is excreted from the ejaculatory ducts. These secretions help keep the spermatozoa alive and aid their passage.[1] Mucous secretions from the bulbourethral glands join the other fluid in the urethra.

The penis contains the urethra surrounded by the right and left corpus cavernosum and the corpus spongiosum urethra. These sponge-like bodies are in the shape of a shaft covered with loosely attached skin and an expanded tip called the glans penis. The glans penis is covered with a doubly folded layer of skin called the prepuce or foreskin. The penis is suspended from the pubic symphysis by suspensory ligaments. A vast network of channels in the cavernosum and spongiosum fill with blood during an erection.

Surgery on any of these structures of the genitourinary system can be performed for diagnostic, reconstructive purposes, or for suspected malignant or instruments for pelvic applications and specialist instruments for retracting the prostate or for grasping and extracting calculi.

Open prostatectomy

An open prostatectomy is the excision and removal of the prostate gland via an abdominal or perineal incision. Open prostatectomy will be performed if the prostate is too large, the age and medical condition of the patient are an acceptable risk, the location of the pathologic condition and presence of associated medical disease suggest this is the best approach, or if the patient cannot attain a lithotomy position. The prostate gland can be removed via three approaches.

- Suprapubic prostatectomy: benign hypertrophic prostatic tissue is removed via a transvesical approach.
- Retropubic prostatectomy: benign or malignant prostatic tissue is removed via an extravesical approach.
- Perineal prostatectomy: prostatic adenoma is removed via a perineal approach.

A perineal prostatectomy will not be described for the purposes of this discussion. The supra- or retropubic prostatectomy patient is positioned in a supine position with slight Trendelenburg and with the legs slightly abducted. The patient is prepared with an antimicrobial solution from above the umbilicus to mid-thigh and laterally to the bedline. The operation can be performed through a low paramedian incision, but is mostly performed through a lower transverse or Pfannenstiel incision.

After the transverse incision is made for a retropubic prostatectomy, the anterior rectus sheath and portions of the internal and external oblique muscles are incised. The rectus abdominis muscles are separated in the midline and retracted laterally to expose the space of Retzius.[1] The anterior portion of the prostatic capsule is incised transversely after traction sutures have been placed. Using either sharp or finger dissection, the surgeon enucleates the prostatic gland from its surgical capsule. Haemostasis is maintained with absorbable sutures and diathermy, then a Foley catheter is inserted via the urethra into the bladder and inflated. The prostatic capsule incision is closed with an interrupted or continuous absorbable

suture. A drain is placed in the space of Retzius and the abdominal wound closed in layers.

For a suprapubic prostatectomy, the entrance into the space of Retzius is as for a retropubic prostatectomy. The surgeon places two traction sutures at either end of the proposed incision line in the dome of the bladder. The incision is made into the bladder and the contents of the bladder are aspirated. The bladder is inspected and then an incision is made in the prostatic mucosa. The surgeon then enucleates the diseased prostate from its cavity using finger dissection. Haemostasis is attained using absorbable sutures. The bladder may be drained at this time with a suprapubic catheter placed through a small stab incision near the suprapubic incision. A Foley catheter with a 30-ml balloon is inserted via the urethra and inflated sufficiently to prevent it falling into the prostatic fossa. The cystectomy incision is closed with two layers of absorbable sutures. A drain is placed in the space of Retzius and the abdominal wound closed in layers.

Nephrectomy

A nephrectomy is the partial or total surgical removal of the kidney. A nephrectomy is indicated for severe renal diseases such as severe hydronephrosis, renal tumours, pyelonephritis, renal artery stenosis, trauma, or calculous disease with infection. Severe diseases of the kidneys often involve the ureters and these are often excised as well.

The patient will be positioned in either the lateral position with the loin over the kidney rest and the operative site uppermost or in a supine position with a sandbag under the back or hip. In the lateral position, the patient's back will be brought closer to the edge of the operating table on the surgeon's side and both arms are supported in a flexed position by arm supports. The lower leg will be flexed and the upper leg extended and supported by a pillow between the legs. The kidney rest is elevated and when the desired degree of bed flexion is obtained, the patient will be secured in position by large adhesive tape. The patient is prepared with antimicrobial solution from the axilla to the ilium and laterally to the bedline. The operation can be performed through a flank, lumbar or thoracoabdominal incision.

A curved incision is made across the flank and the skin, fat and fascia are incised with haemostasis being

V   **Trigeminal nerve**: (1) sensory supply to forehead, eyes, meninges, face, jaw, teeth, hard palate, buccal mucosa, tongue, nose, nasal mucosa and maxillary sinus and (2) motor innervation of the muscles of mastication.

VI   **Abducens nerve**: motor nerve to lateral rectus muscle of eye.

VII   **Facial nerve**: supplies the musculature of the face and the anterior two-thirds of the tongue.

VIII   **Acoustic nerve**: sensory nerve for the cochlear for hearing and the vestibular for balance.

IX   **Glossopharyngeal**: supplies the sense of taste for posterior third of tongue and sensation to the tonsils and pharyngeal region and partially innervates the pharyngeal muscles.

X   **Vagus nerve**: motor and sensory functions, innervation of pharyngeal and laryngeal musculature, control of heart rate, regulation of acid secretion of the stomach.

XI   **Spinal accessory**: motor nerve to the sternocleidomastoid and trapezius muscles.

XII   **Hypoglossal nerve**: innervates the musculature of the tongue.[1]

A way to remember the names of the cranial nerves is given in Table 8.1

The spinal nerves have no special names but the 31 pairs are numbered according to the level of the spinal column at which they exit. There are eight cervical pairs, 12 thoracic, five lumbar, five sacral and one coccygeal. Each nerve attaches to the spinal column by means of two short roots, the dorsal root and the ventral root. The dorsal or posterior root generally leads nerve fibres from the sensory receptors to various areas of the body, while the ventral or anterior root motor nerve fibre is supplying voluntary and involuntary muscles and glands. The large branches of each spinal nerve form networks called plexuses that distribute branches to the various body parts.[2] The three main plexuses are the cervical plexuses, the brachial plexuses and the lumbosacral plexuses.

Neurosurgical procedures can be performed to diagnose or resect pathological lesions, to relieve pressure on the brain or spinal cord related to disease or injury, or to relieve pressure or repair peripheral nerves.

Perioperative nursing considerations

Patients undergoing cranial neurosurgical procedures often experience extreme anxiety related to their surgical outcome. The onset of symptoms is frequently sudden and psychologically the patient has difficulty accepting the relationship between their diagnosis and their symptoms. Patients, both male and female, are apprehensive about the removal of their hair for craniotomy and the reaction from their friends. Their wishes concerning partial or complete hair removal should be complied with if possible.

In planning for the specific needs of the patient, the nurse will identify the following areas for consideration.

- The appropriate positioning of the patient to prevent pressure areas. These patients may have compromised sensation and mobility to affected areas of their body.
- The size of the patient may necessitate extra equipment for safe positioning, and extra personnel may be necessary for safe transferring onto the operating table.
- The scrub nurse will need a thorough knowledge of the specialist procedures required for neurosurgery.
- The scrub nurse will need a good knowledge of the positions required for neurosurgical procedures.

Table 8.1 **Cranial nerves: a way to remember their names in order**	
Old	olfactory
Oscar	optic
Often	occulomotor
Tried	trochlear
Taking	trigeminal
A	abducens
Fine	facial
Australian	acoustic
Golden	glossopharyngeal
Vintage	vagus
After	accessory
Hours	hypoglossal

- All scans, X-rays and appropriate tests should be available in the operating theatre.
- Specialist equipment such as the operating microscope, fibreoptic headlight and powered drills should be available.
- A shave tray and clippers, marking pen and local anaesthetic should be available for cleaning, shaving, marking and infiltrating the proposed incision line on the head immediately before surgery.
- A urinary catheter may be inserted before surgery.
- Suction and diathermy equipment should be tested and ready.
- Assessment of sensory deficits such as hearing and sight in the elderly patient.

SURGICAL INTERVENTIONS

Neurosurgical operations can be performed either on the cranium, the spine or on the peripheral nerves. Cranial surgery is performed by opening the bony cranial cavity to gain access to the brain and supporting structures. Cranial neurosurgical procedures are mostly performed to relieve pressure on the brain due to injury or disease, to remove pathological tumours or lesions, or to create a diversionary pathway for CSF to reduce pressure caused by excess fluid accumulation. The most common procedures are burr holes, craniotomy and ventriculoperitoneal shunt.

Spinal neurosurgical procedures are performed to remove tumours or lesions from the spinal cord, to reduce severe pain, or to replace or reinforce injured and diseased vertebral discs. Commonly performed spinal procedures are laminectomy and anterior cervical fusion.

Peripheral neurosurgical procedures are performed to repair partially or fully severed peripheral nerves, for diagnostic procedures, or for relieving severe pain caused by pressure from surrounding structures. The most commonly performed operation on peripheral nerves is the carpal tunnel release for carpal tunnel syndrome.

Cranial procedures

For cranial procedures, the patient will be positioned either in a supine position with the head rotated to give access to frontal and temporal regions, or laterally in a 'park bench' position to gain access to the temporal and posterior regions. Not as commonly used are the prone and sitting, or upright, positions for access to the posterior fossa regions. For the procedures described, the patient will be positioned in the supine position with the head positioned either in a Mayfield horseshoe-shaped head support, or with a Mayfield pin headrest attached. Immediately before surgery, the patient's head is fully or partially shaved with clippers then with a razor, the incision line is marked with an indelible pen and then infiltrated with local anaesthetic as a vasoconstrictor. Special care is taken to ensure the eyes are protected from pressure and covered to prevent corneal abrasions and contamination with prepping solution.

Burr holes/craniotomy

Burr holes are holes drilled through the skull to expose the structures beneath. These are the simplest of cranial openings and are usually performed to evacuate a haematoma that has accumulated in or on brain tissue. Intracranial haematomas are classified as extradural, subdural or intercerebral depending on the location of the involved pathology. Extradural haematomas form when the middle meningeal artery is torn and forms a haematoma between the skull and the dura. This is an acute emergency and requires immediate surgical intervention. Subdural haematomas form between the dura and the arach-

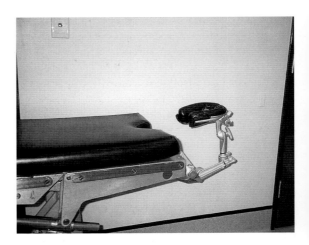

Fig. 8.22 Cranial headrest

intractable pain caused by advanced stages of some diseases and (3) to remove tumours of the nerve sheath and nerve cells.[2] One of the most common peripheral nerve operations is for carpal tunnel syndrome.

Carpal tunnel release

A carpal tunnel release is a decompression of the median nerve on the volar surface of the wrist. This operation is performed to relieve the symptoms of numbness, tingling of fingers and weakness of intrinsic thumb muscles caused by compression of the median nerve by the transverse carpal ligament or by displacement of the lunate bone or volar carpal ganglion.[1]

The patient is positioned in a supine position with the affected arm on a hand table and the other arm either on an armboard or by their side. A tourniquet is applied to the upper affected arm. This operation may be performed under local, regional or general anaesthesia.

A longitudinal skin incision is made paralleling the thenar palm crease. The wound is retracted with small hand held retractors or a small self-retaining retractor. A haemostat is introduced at the proximal end, pointing towards the distal end, of the carpal ligament and spread open. The carpal ligament is then incised over the haemostat that is protecting the median nerve. The wound is closed with fine nylon sutures and dressed with a bulky dressing of sheet wool and possibly a splint.

THORACIC SURGERY

Thoracic surgery involves procedures on the structures of the pulmonary system. The pulmonary system consists of the skeletal framework of the thorax, the pleural cavity containing a pair of lungs surrounded by a membrane called the pleura, and the mediastinal cavity which encloses a portion of the trachea, the right and left bronchi, blood vessels, lymph nodes and nerves.

The skeletal framework of the thorax is formed posteriorly by 12 thoracic vertebrae, laterally by 12 pairs of ribs and anteriorly by the sternum and costal cartilages. Posteriorly the 12 pairs of ribs articulate with their corresponding thoracic vertebrae. Anteriorly, the upper part of the sternum (manubrium) articulates with the clavicles and the first two ribs, the

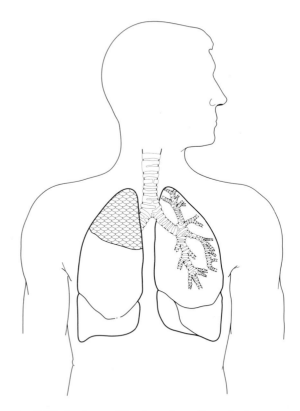

Fig. 8.28 Anatomy of the thoracic cavity contents

body (gladiolus) articulates with ribs three through seven, whilst the eighth, ninth and tenth ribs articulate with the costal cartilages of the rib above and the eleventh and twelfth are not attached anteriorly. The lower sternum is called the xiphoid process and is fused to the gladiolus in early development. Filling the spaces between the ribs are the internal and external intercostal muscles, arteries, veins and nerves.

The right and left pleural cavity are lined by a membrane called the parietal pleura which covers the cavity posteriorly on the inner surfaces of the ribs and the mediastinum medially and the surface of the diaphragm. At the root of the lungs the membrane is reflected back to cover the lungs and the lining is now called visceral pleura. A serous secretion called pleural fluid provides lubrication between these two membranes to minimise friction.[1]

The lungs extend from their apex at the base of the neck to the diaphragm and are the essential organs of respiration.[1] The right lung is divided into an upper, inserted and the ribs closed with strong sutures. The wound is closed in layers and the drains connected to an underwater sealed drainage system.

When a lobectomy is required, the affected lung is exposed through a posterolateral thoracotomy incision as for the procedure for a thoracotomy. The visceral pleura around the hilum is dissected free, and the branches of the pulmonary artery, pulmonary veins and the bronchus connected to the diseased lobe are identified, isolated, clamped, double ligated or stapled, and divided. The fissure between the affected lobe and the connecting lobe is dissected free if adhesions exist. The staple and suture lines are tested for air leaks, the cavity irrigated with normal saline and haemostasis attained. Chest drains are inserted and connected to an underwater sealed drainage system. The wound is closed as for a pneumonectomy.

For a segmental resection of the lung, the affected segment of lung is exposed as for a thoracotomy. The pleura is incised from the affected segment and the segmental artery, veins and bronchus are identified, isolated, clamped, ligated or stapled, and divided. The bronchus of the affected segment needs to be clamped and the remaining lung inflated to ensure the affected segment is confirmed and the clamp properly placed before division. The affected segment is removed by dissection from the remaining segments. The suture/staple lines are tested for air leaks, the cavity irrigated with normal saline, and haemostasis attained. Chest drains are inserted and connected to an underwater sealed drainage system. The wound is closed as for a pneumonectomy.

VASCULAR SURGERY

Vascular surgery involves procedures on the peripheral vascular system, which is a vast complex network of vessels whose major function is to transport blood and vital substances to all parts of the body.

The system consists of arteries that carry blood away from the heart, and veins that carry blood to the heart. Arteries and veins consist of three layers: the fibrous outer layer (tunica adventitia), a muscular middle layer (tunica media) and a smooth inner layer (tunica intima). Arteries have a thick muscle layer and can contract, whereas veins have a thin muscle layer and valves that prevent backflow. Both veins and arteries are regulated by the autonomic nervous system. The arterial system carrying oxygenated blood from the heart via the greatest vessel, the aorta, branches many times into progressively smaller vessels until the smallest tubules called capillaries reach the cellular level. At the cellular level, an exchange of nutrients and metabolic waste is achieved between the arterioles and venules, then the venules, the smallest of the veins carrying deoxygenated blood, become progressively larger until the veins form the vena cava, which re-enters the heart.

Blood flow depends on viscosity, vessel wall resistance and the peripheral resistance of the arterioles, and disruption in any of these factors reduces the vessel's ability to transport blood effectively. When a significant disruption occurs and the systemic perfusion is compromised, surgical intervention is necessary.

Perioperative nursing considerations

For patients undergoing vascular surgery, a nursing assessment should involve the routine questions with special attention given to physical conditions associated with circulatory problems. These problems may be compounded by associated medical conditions of poor circulation such as cardiac, renal, pulmonary diseases, diabetes and clotting problems. The population requiring interventions for vascular procedures will include an increasing population of the elderly. These patients may have a variety of physiological impairments and provision will need to be made to accommodate these in the operative stages. Poor lifestyle habits of diet and smoking may have been a contributing causative factor, and the perioperative nurse should ensure her questions and attitudes are non-judgmental in nature.

There are other possible nursing considerations.

- Observation of general physical appearance to assess skin integrity especially in the elderly.
- Assessment of the effects of vascular disease such as muscle and skin atrophy, tissue ulceration or necrosis, changes in skin colour, and pain.
- Assessment of sensory deficits such as hearing.

- Any previous problems with anaesthesia.
- Ensuring any X-rays, angiograms and studies are present in the theatre for review.
- An assessment of the size of the patient may identify a need for longer surgical instruments.
- Observation of any limitations in mobility, such as neck stiffness or limited hip movements.
- Identification of the correct side of the body for surgery.
- Ensure methods of keeping the patient warm are available, as vascular surgery can be lengthy and the patient is already peripherally cold.

SURGICAL INTERVENTION

Vascular surgical procedures involving the peripheral vascular system are mainly performed on the large vessels to improve systemic circulation and tissue perfusion throughout the body. This improvement can be achieved by incising the vessel and removing the obstruction (endarterectomy or thrombectomy) or by bypassing the area of disease with a graft. The main vascular surgical procedures are the abdominal aortic aneurysm repair, the femoropopliteal bypass graft or the carotid endarterectomy. For each vascular procedure the patient may be heparinised before clamping the vessels to begin the repairs and reversed with protamine sulphate after the anastomoses are complete.

Abdominal aortic aneurysm repair

An aortic aneurysm repair is the excision and/or internal bypass of an aneurysm of the wall of the abdominal aorta using the insertion of an internal synthetic graft to re-establish vascular continuity. An aneurysm is a sac caused by the dilatation of a weakened wall of the vessel. The major causes of an aortic aneurysm are arteriosclerotic disease, infection or trauma. They can be asymptomatic and diagnosed when other diseases are being investigated, especially coronary artery disease, or when the patient presents with the symptoms of severe back pain, hypotension, shock and distal vascular insufficiency when rupture has occurred. When this emergency occurs, the prime consideration is the control of haemorrhage at the point of rupture, but other risks

involved are injury to the ureters, renal failure, spinal cord ischaemia and death.[1]

The patient is placed in a supine position with the arms extended on armboards. The skin is prepared as for abdominal procedures from the nipple line to mid-thigh and laterally to the bedline with an antimicrobial solution. The abdomen is opened through a midline incision from the xiphoid process to the symphysis pubis. An exploratory laparotomy is conducted and a self-retaining retractor inserted. The intestines are mobilised and some are lifted out of the abdominal cavity and wrapped in a moist abdominal scarf to give better exposure.

The peritoneum is incised over the aorta and extended superiorly and inferiorly to expose the aorta above the aneurysm, and the bifurcation below. The patient is heparinised and being careful to avoid the renal arteries and ureters, an aortic vascular clamp is placed across the aorta and closed. The aneurysm is opened and the thrombotic and atheromatous material shelled out and removed. The aneurysm wall is left to provide a covering for the graft. The prosthetic graft is chosen according to the surgeon's preference and the size of the aorta and is prepared as per the manufacturer's instructions. The graft is anastomosed to the prepared proximal aorta with continuous through-and-through double-armed vascular sutures. The repair is irrigated continuously with heparinised saline to keep the suture line clean from blood and debris and to allow better visualisation. A clamp is placed lower down the graft and the upper vascular clamp on the aorta eased open to fill the graft with blood and to check the suture line for leaks. If a bifurcated graft is used, the femoral/iliac vessels are inspected for plaque, cleaned and tested for back bleeding. Each side of the graft is anastomosed to the appropriate vessel using the same technique and a smaller double-armed vascular suture. After the first side has been anastomosed, blood is slowly allowed to circulate with the unattached limb of the graft being clamped to prevent leakage. On completion, suture lines are checked for leakage, then the aneurysm sac is trimmed and closed over the graft. The patient's heparinisation is reversed with protamine sulphate. The peritoneum is closed and the intestines returned to their anatomical position and the abdominal wound closed in the routine manner.

Each half of the heart contains an upper and lower communicating chamber. The upper chambers or atria are the receiving chambers: the right atrium receives desaturated blood from the inferior and superior vena cava and the left atrium receives oxygenated blood from the left and right pulmonary veins. Blood blows from the atria through the atrioventricular valves into the ventricles. The pumping chambers or ventricles pump blood into the pulmonary circulatory system via the pulmonary artery from the right side and to the body's systemic circulatory system via the aorta from the left side.

The four valves of the heart consist of two atrioventricular and two semilunar valves. The atrioventricular valves include the tricuspid, which separates the right atrium and right ventricle, and the mitral valve, which separates the left atrium and the left ventricle. The semilunar valves include the pulmonary valve, located between the pulmonary artery and right ventricle, and the aortic valve, located between the left ventricle and the aorta. These valves are designed to maintain forward blood flow and to prevent regurgitation into the originating chamber.

The **left and right coronary arteries** supply oxygen and nutrients to the heart. These originate in the aortic root immediately above the aortic valve in the ascending aorta. The right main coronary artery runs in a groove between the right atrium and right ventricle and branches to the left ventricle (marginal branch of the right coronary artery). The left main coronary artery bifurcates soon after its origin into the circumflex branch of the left coronary artery and the left anterior descending coronary artery. The circumflex coronary artery passes to the back of the heart dividing into a main branch known as the marginal branch of the circumflex coronary artery. The left anterior descending coronary artery provides most of the left ventricle's blood supply.

The **aortic root** is the proximal portion of the aorta containing a fibrous ring called the annulus that encircles the aorta. From the annulus are suspended the cusps of the aortic valve behind which the vessel wall forms the sinuses of Valsalva from which originate the coronary arteries. These sinuses are pouch-like openings that dilate when the aortic valve opens, thus preventing the cusps of the valve obstructing the flow of blood into the coronary arteries. The **aortic arch** is the portion of the aorta from the ascending aorta to the beginning of the descending aorta. Three main vessels branching from the arch are the brachiocephalic or innominate artery, the left common carotid artery and the left subclavian artery.

The **internal mammary arteries** lie behind and parallel to the lateral borders of the sternum. They are used during coronary artery surgery as either a pedicle graft with its own blood supply or as a free graft. The left internal mammary artery has enough length to be used as a pedicle graft and will attach directly to the left anterior descending coronary artery. The right internal mammary artery is shorter and is used as a free graft.

Perioperative nursing considerations

For patients undergoing cardiac surgery, a nursing assessment should involve the routine questions with special attention given to physical conditions associated with cardiac and circulatory problems.

The population requiring interventions for cardiac procedures will include an increasing population of the elderly. These patients may have a variety of physiological impairments and provision will need to be made to accommodate these in the operative stages. Poor lifestyle habits of diet and smoking may have been a contributing causative factor, and the

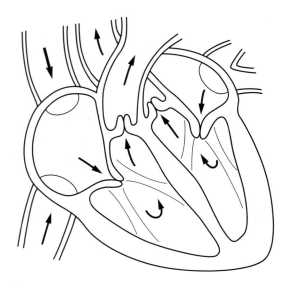

Fig. 8.34 Anatomy of the heart: coronary blood flow

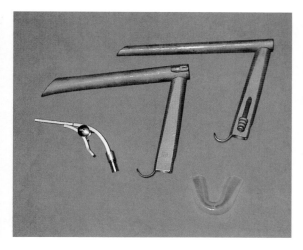

Fig. 8.48 Laryngoscope

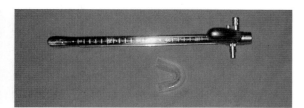

Fig. 8.49 Oesophagoscope

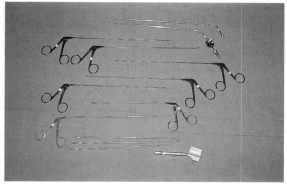

Fig. 8.50 Microlaryngoscopy instruments

Microlaryngoscopy

A microlaryngoscopy is visualisation of the larynx using the laryngoscope and the operating microscope. This procedure is used when the surgeon needs to perform minor procedures on the larynx such as removing polyps or nodes from the vocal cords, or when the laser is used.

The patient is positioned as for a panendoscopy.

The laryngoscope is inserted into the side of the patient's mouth and directed toward the midline, the dorsum of the tongue is elevated and the epiglottis is exposed. The laryngoscope is attached to the self-retaining laryngoscope holder positioned on a Mayo table placed over the patient's chest. The microscope is positioned, then the larynx and vocal cords are examined and biopsies are taken, or the polyps or nodes stripped off the vocal cords. The scrub nurse must place the instruments and suction tube into the hand of the surgeon and direct the closed tips into the entrance of the laryngoscope.

If the laser is to be used then all laser precautions as described in the section on laser must be followed. A laser safety officer must be added to the theatre's staff. The patient's face and eyes must be protected with moist drapes to prevent accidental injury. The laser may be used to destroy tissue at a precise point with minimal destruction of the surrounding tissue. It is used to destroy vocal papillomas, and carcinoma *in situ* of the larynx and for some endobronchial lesions.[1] Instruments for laser surgery are the same as for microlaryngoscopy but the instruments should be ebonised. A self-retaining laryngoscope holder and the microscope with the micromanipulator attached to the head needs to be added to the equipment prepared. A smoke evacuator is necessary for the evacuation of surgical plume. Commercially prepared laser-retardant endotracheal tubes and a jet ventilation system are necessary for intubation. Care must be taken to keep all areas of the patient in the operative area covered with moist drapes and pads. Sterile normal saline and a filled syringe must be kept on the set-up in case of fire. The laser safety officer must ensure all theatre personnel wear the personal protective equipment provided, that the theatre has laser signs posted and entrance to the theatre is restricted.

The operative procedure is as for a microlaryngoscopy with the additional use by the surgeon of the laser.

Uvulopalatopharyngoplasty (UPPP)

A UPPP is the removal of a portion of the soft palate including the tonsils and the uvula. This operation is performed to relieve obstructive sleep apnoea and snoring.

The patient is positioned in a supine position with the neck hyperextended by placing a sandbag under the shoulders. A mouth gag (usually a Boyle–Davis tonsil gag with blades) is positioned. The tissue to be resected may be outlined with the diathermy then incised with a sharp knife and toothed tissue forceps. The incision extends from anterior to the tonsillar pillar up and across the soft palate above the uvula and down to include the tonsillar pillar on the opposite side. The tissue may be resected with long Metzenbaum scissors and a toothed forceps or with the electrosurgical pencil. Haemostasis is maintained by the electrosurgical pencil. The mucosal edges are sutured with a continuous absorbable suture. The operative site should be irrigated and suctioned to clear away debris and to check for haemostasis. This procedure may also be performed using the laser.

Tonsillectomy

A tonsillectomy is the excision of the palatine tonsils and, if necessary, the adenoids (nasopharyngeal tonsils). This procedure is performed to relieve symptoms associated with chronic tonsillitis and otitis media, and nasal obstruction due to enlarged adenoid glands.

The patient is positioned in a supine position with slight Trendelenburg. The neck is slightly hyperextended by placing a small sandbag or rolled towel under the patient's shoulders.

A self-retaining retractor is placed to retract the mouth open (usually a Boyle–Davis mouth gag with blades). A tonsil is grasped with a tonsil-grasping forceps and an incision made in the mucous membrane of the anterior pillar. The tissue is freed from its attachments with a tonsil dissector preserving the posterior tonsil pillar. A tonsil snare is then looped over the tonsil and snapped over the pillar releasing the tonsil. The fossa is packed with a gauze pack or tonsil sponge to aid haemostasis whilst the other tonsil is removed. Haemostasis is attained with the use of a diathermy forceps or with absorbable ligatures. The adenoids are removed with an adenoid curette either before or after the tonsillectomy. Care should be taken to have suction available at all times during and after the procedure. The patient should

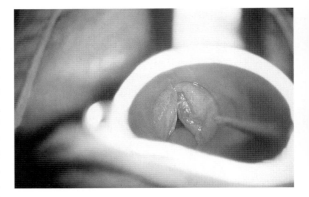

Fig. 8.51 Cancer of the larynx

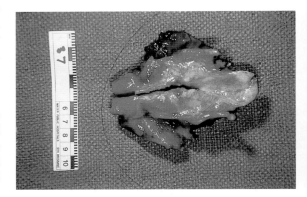

Fig. 8.52 Larynx after removal

be positioned on their side to aid the drainage of secretion before leaving the theatre.

Laryngectomy

A total laryngectomy is the complete removal of the cartilaginous larynx, the hyoid bone and the strap muscles connected to the larynx. This procedure is performed to remove tumours of the larynx and hypolarynx. If the cancer has metastasised to surrounding nodes then a radical neck dissection will be performed as well.

The patient is placed in a supine position with the neck slightly extended by placing the shoulders on a rolled towel or small gel log. The patient is intubated with a reinforced endotracheal tube. The neck is prepared with antimicrobial solution from the jaw line to nipple line and to the bed line laterally.

A midline incision is made from the suprasternal notch to the crease of the neck. The skin flaps are elevated on each side and retracted away from the operative site. The strap muscles (sternothyroid, sternohyoid, omohyoid) are divided in the midline and retracted. The suprahyoid muscles are divided from the hyoid bone and the bone is divided after the first lateral third with bone-cutting forceps. The superior laryngeal nerve and vessels are dissected out, divided and ligated. The midline of the thyroid gland is incised and the gland and vessels dissected laterally off the trachea. The inferior pharyngeal constrictor muscle is severed from its attachment to the thyroid cartilage on each side.[1]

The trachea is transected below the cricoid cartilage with care being taken not to damage the oesophagus. The cartilage's inferior edge is grabbed with a grasping tissue forceps and held upwards while another cuffed reinforced endotracheal tube is positioned in the trachea. The larynx is retracted upwards whilst it is dissected free from the cervical oesophagus. The pharynx is entered above the epiglottis and incised down to meet the lateral excision of the larynx. The specimen is removed and a moist sponge placed in the wound.

The tracheostomy stoma is fashioned and a tracheostomy tube inserted and ventilation is re-established. A nasogastric tube is inserted and guided into the oesophagus. The pharyngeal and oesophageal defect is closed with fine absorbable sutures in two layers. The muscles and thyroid are sutured into place with interrupted sutures. Suction drains are placed and the wound is closed in layers.

Radical neck dissection

A radical neck dissection is the removal of the lymphatic chain and all non-vital structures of the neck. A neck dissection may be performed at the same time as removal of the primary cancer or later if metastasis occurs. The primary tumour may be in the oropharynx, a cutaneous malignant melanoma or advanced skin cancer in the head and neck region. Neck dissections may be performed with reconstruction planned. Therefore, preservation of as much local flap material as possible will be taken into account when mapping the initial incision lines.

The patient will be positioned in a supine position with slight extension of the neck and slight Trendelenburg. The area to be prepared with antimicrobial solution will depend on the extent of the tumour involvement and the proposed flap or graft sites. For a radical neck dissection with no reconstruction, the patient will be prepared from above the ear, across the mandibular jaw line anteriorly, down to the nipple line and laterally to the bed line including the shoulder. For tumours involving the mouth, the opening into the oral cavity will need to be included in the preparation. The graft sites may include the abdomen for a free jejunal graft, a forearm for a free radial artery graft, the chest for a pectoralis major musculocutaneous free flap or deltopectoral pedicle flap or the thigh for a skin graft.

No specific incision line can be used to treat all neck dissections, therefore the incision will vary according to the type of resection and reconstruction planned. After a 'Y' incision has been performed through the skin and platysma, the upper flap will be retracted upwards and the flaps dissected from the vertical incision line will be retracted laterally. The dissection will include the removal of all lymph-bearing tissue from the midline anteriorly to the trapezius muscle posteriorly and from the mandible superiorly to the clavicle inferiorly. The tissue between the deep cervical fascia and the platysma muscle externally is removed except the carotid artery system, the vagus, phrenic and hypoglossal nerves, and the brachial plexus. The non-vital structures removed on the side of the neck with the tumour are the jugular vein, eleventh cranial nerve, sternocleidomastoid muscle and the submandibular salivary gland. The surgical specimen is removed en masse. The surgical field is irrigated with warm saline and examined for bleeding. A tracheostomy will be performed in all radical neck dissections and a prophylactic tracheostomy may be performed in simple neck dissections if respiratory distress is anticipated. Suction drains are placed to protect viability of the thin skin flaps and facilitate approximation of wound surfaces. The subcutaneous tissue is sutured with absorbable sutures, then the wound edges are approximated with non-absorbable sutures or skin staples.

Reconstructive procedures may be performed after head and neck procedures have removed malignant tumours to correct surgical defects and restore function. The type of reconstruction will depend on the site of the defect. The reconstructive surgery may involve teams of plastic and general surgeons as well as the ear, nose and throat (ENT) surgeons. Regional flaps (such as the **pectoralis major** myocutaneous pedicle flap) may be used to reconstruct the floor of the mouth. A free jejunal flap or radial artery forearm flap may be used to restore continuity of the oropharynx and restore defects. If part of the mandibular is resected, a vascularised bone graft from a rib or the iliac crest may be used to restore the functions of speech and chewing. The microvascular flaps will extend surgical time significantly as vessels will need to be anastomosed microscopically and bone grafts may need to be fixated with plates and screws.

PLASTIC AND RECONSTRUCTIVE SURGERY

Plastic surgery involves procedures that restore and correct defects and deformities to all parts of the body and achieve cosmetic improvement. Cosmetic plastic surgery can be performed for cosmetic correction that may or may not be related to the physical health of the patient. Reconstructive plastic surgery is usually performed when traumatic injury causes disfigurement or to correct congenital abnormalities.

Plastic surgery treatment can be categorised into four main problem areas.[2]

- Repair of traumatic injuries to reconstruct and restore function and improve body appearance, e.g. burns and facial injuries.
- Resection of benign and malignant tumours that leave soft tissue defects.
- Correction of congenital abnormalities, especially in children.
- Improvement of appearance, e.g. breast enhancement or reduction.

This section will cover adult surgery only. See the chapter on children's surgery for correction of congenital abnormalities.

Perioperative nursing considerations

For patients undergoing plastic and reconstructive surgery, a nursing assessment should involve the routine questions to obtain an accurate nursing and medical history. Special attention should be given to physical conditions associated with the problems that have brought the patient to surgery. For example, if the patient's admission is the result of road trauma, then there may be other major injuries that need to be considered during positioning. These patients may experience major alterations to their body image as limbs and faces may have been severely damaged. The population requiring interventions for plastic and reconstructive procedures will include both children and young and old adults. Many patients will be fit and healthy adults undergoing cosmetic surgery but will be experiencing anxiety related to their surgical outcome.

There are other possible nursing considerations.

- Observation of general physical appearance to assess skin integrity especially in the elderly.
- Any previous problems with anaesthesia. Drug reactions to local anaesthetic should be noted as these agents may be used extensively during this surgery.
- Ensuring any X-rays, scans, consultations with other surgeons and any other studies are present in the theatre for review.
- Observation of any limitations in mobility.
- Advise the patient undergoing rhinological procedures that they will have a nasal pack inserted postoperatively.
- Advise these patients that they may experience alterations in the senses of smell and taste postoperatively.
- Advise patients that they may still have visible suture lines but they will fade with time.

SURGICAL INTERVENTIONS

A wide variety of operations are standard practice in plastic and reconstructive surgery. These operations are not limited to a single anatomical or biological system or to a single operative technique but are inclusive of basic and specialist techniques. Some of the specialist techniques may include microvascular free flaps or reimplantation of limbs and digits to restore functional use of a body part. Some of the more common cosmetic procedures may be rhinoplasty (described in rhinological procedures), reduction mammoplasty, augmentation mammoplasty, and rhytidectomy (facelift). The most common reconstruction surgery may be skin grafting (full and partial thickness), reduction of facial fractures, breast reconstruction. It should be noted that very fine instruments, sutures and frequent use of the surgical scalpel are employed to give clean skin edges and good approximation for fast healing and minimal scarring.

Skin grafts (full and partial thickness)

A free skin graft provides an effective method of covering a wound if infection is absent, haemostasis is achieved and vascularity is adequate. Skin from the donor site is removed and transplanted to the recipient site where it develops vascular viability from the capillary ingrowth from the wound bed. Soft tissue autografts are preferred because of compatible skin colour and texture to the area of tissue being replaced. The thickness of the graft can be either partial or full thickness.

Partial-thickness grafts contain epidermis and only a portion of the dermis from the donor site. These are used to cover large denuded areas on surfaces such as the back, trunk and legs.

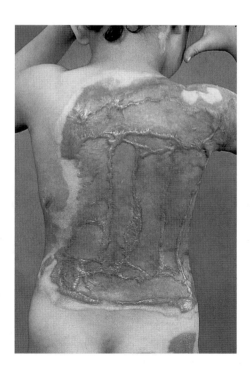

Fig. 8.53 Skin grafting to burns

The patient is positioned so that both donor and recipient sites are exposed and can be prepared and draped. The recipient site is prepared, which might involve removal of scar tissue, eschar, wound debridement, or removal of a benign or malignant tumour. An estimate of the size of the skin graft required is made. The depth of the graft is calibrated on the dermatome or skin-grafting knife. The graft is harvested and kept moist in normal saline-soaked sponges until required. The donor site is covered with zeroform-impregnated gauze and a combine and wrapped. If bleeding needs to be controlled, then adrenaline and saline-soaked sponges are placed over the graft site until haemostasis is maintained. If the graft is to be meshed, it is applied to the carrier selected for the size required and meshed. Meshing produces multiple uniform slits in the skin graft, which allows for the expansion of multiple apertures in the graft for drainage and extends the skin over a greater area. The graft is applied to the recipient site and may be left unattached, stapled or sutured. A non-adherent dressing may be applied first and then dressings as per the surgeon's preference. A balance must be maintained in the amount of pressure applied by dressings as enough is required to make the graft adhere, but too much pressure will damage the delicate cellular structures.

Full-thickness grafts contain epidermis and dermis greater than a depth of 1 mm. The advantage of this type of graft is that it does not contract very much in size and can be used in areas of flexion, where there has been a loss or padding is required, and it has a greater ability to withstand trauma.[1] It is preferred for the face, neck, hands, elbows, knees and axilla.

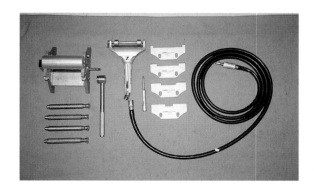

Fig. 8.54 Dermatome and a skin mesher

Perioperative care of adults

If a full-thickness graft is taken, fat adherent to the graft is trimmed and the graft applied to the recipient site. The graft is usually sutured at the edges with the suture ends left long to tie over a pressure dressing. If the skin is not to be laid immediately, it is kept moist with saline-soaked sponges until it is prepared for preservation. The skin is gently flattened, smoothed out and placed on moist saline-soaked fine gauze with the skin side downwards. It is then folded loosely and placed in a sterile jar. The jar is labelled with the patient's details and placed in a refrigerator until required.

Flaps (pedicle flap and free flap)

Flaps that carry their own blood supply are usually used to cover recipient sites that have poor vascularity and full-thickness tissue loss where reconstruction or wound closure is desired. Flaps are classified according to their blood supply (random pattern, axial pattern), or to their position or how they are rotated after elevation (advancement, transposition, rotation, island, pedicle). Flaps can also be free flaps where autotransplantation of tissue is involved.

A pedicle flap remains attached at one or both ends of the donor site during transfer to the recipient site. The vascular supply is maintained from vessels in the pedicle. A free flap is the removal of tissue including the vascular bundle to the recipient site where the vessels are anastomosed to recipient vessels to re-establish vascularity.

The patient is positioned, prepared and draped as for a skin graft. The recipient site is prepared to take the flap by incision and removal of the tumour or debridement of the area. An assessment is made of the size and shape of the flap required. The donor site will have been decided before surgery. The flap is incised, elevated and transferred to the recipient site where the edges are sutured to the periphery of the recipient site. If a free flap has been taken, microvascular anastomoses to the vessels prepared at the recipient site will be performed. The flap donor site is repaired by direct closure or by covering the defect with a skin graft or both. A drain may be placed under the recipient flap and the donor site dressed. The recipient site may or may not be dressed as they are often left exposed so that vascu-

larity of the flap may be easily checked and recorded and pressure is not applied to the delicate vascular structures.

Reduction mammoplasty

A reduction mammoplasty is the removal of excess breast and skin tissue with reconstruction of the remaining breast tissue. A reduction mammoplasty is performed to alleviate symptoms associated with heavy, pendulous breasts resulting in both physical and psychological problems. Some of the indications for surgery are back pain because of the added weight that constantly pulls the body forward, deep grooving in the shoulders from the weight of the breast, intertrigo or need to achieve symmetry following surgery on the contralateral side after a mastectomy.[1,2]

The patient is positioned in a supine position with the arms slightly extended on armboards on either side. The surgical incision lines and site for the new nipple may be mapped out on the breasts with an indelible marker before prepping or after the skin preparation and care should be taken not to remove the markings. The skin is prepared from the base of the neck to the umbilicus and laterally to the bed line including the axilla area.

The skin between the new and old nipple sites is incised and removed with the nipple remaining attached to the underlying breast tissue as a pedicle. The nipples will be removed and reapplied as free grafts when the reduction is complete in patients with very large breasts. Redundant breast tissue inferior to the nipple is excised through an inverted 'T' incision. Each nipple and the adjacent tissue is mobilised and sutured into place. The tissue removed is weighed and recorded. The medial and lateral skin edges are approximated in a vertical suture line inferior to the nipple. The incision in the inframammary fold is trimmed and closed in a transverse suture line. Suction drains may be placed and the wound dressed in a protective dressing.

Augmentation mammoplasty

An augmentation mammoplasty is the insertion of a saline-filled prosthetic implant behind or under the breast tissue to increase its size. An augmentation mammoplasty is performed for patients whose breasts are smaller than desired, on patients whose breasts are asymmetrical and after a subcutaneous mastectomy.

The patient is positioned in a supine position with the arms extended on armboards. The skin is prepared from the base of the neck to the umbilicus and laterally to the bed line including the axilla area. The procedure may be carried out through an inframammary, periareolar or transaxillary incision. For inframammary insertion, a pocket is developed in the plane between the pectoralis fascia and posterior capsule of the breast. Haemostasis is obtained and the implant inserted. After adjusting the implant to sit correctly, the incision is closed. For periareolar insertion, the incision is made along the inferior border of the areola. The subcutaneous tissue is dissected and the retromammary space enlarged to the appropriate size. After haemostasis is obtained, the prosthesis is inserted and adjusted. The breast tissue and incision is closed according to the surgeon's preference. For transaxillary insertion, a vertical or oblique incision is made in the axilla down through the subcutaneous tissue. A pocket is created over the upper pole of the breast and the prosthesis is inserted. The incision is closed in layers. The breasts are dressed in a protective dressing.

Breast reconstruction

A breast reconstruction is the rebuilding of a breast either with existing tissue and an implant, or tissue expanders and an implant, or with a flap either with or without an implant. Breast reconstruction is performed following mastectomy to restore shape to the breast area and to restore body image psychologically for the patient. This procedure may be performed immediately following the mastectomy or may be delayed.

Using existing tissue is the easiest method but this will depend if sufficient tissue remains after the mastectomy for the procedure. When sufficient tissue remains, an implant of the appropriate size is placed under the remaining skin flap and/or muscle. The opposite side may need to be adjusted by a reduction mammoplasty.

Tissue expansion is stretching normal tissue adjacent to the defect to create redundant skin and tissue to correct the defect. This is achieved in breast reconstruction by placing an expander the same shape as the breast in place and by injecting saline into the attached valve to gradually expand the implant until the tissue has stretched to the desired result. The operative procedure is similar to an augmentation mammoplasty with the additional tunnel and pocket being created to receive the injection dome and connecting tube. The expander is tested for leaks before insertion and expanded with sterile saline solution until blanching of the skin occurs. The gradual expansion will continue over several weeks until the desired stretch is achieved and then the temporary expander is exchanged for a permanent prosthesis.

For procedures where a flap is required to replace a tissue deficit, either a **latissimus dorsi** myocutaneous flap or a **transrectus abdominis** myocutaneous flap can be used. If a latissimus dorsi flap is performed, the patient is positioned laterally so access can be gained to the operative site. The skin island and area of dissection is marked and the skin island incised transversely across the back. The muscle is freed from the overlying surrounding skin by undermining so that part or all of the muscle may be mobilised. The skin island and muscle are transferred from the axilla to the chest wall via a tunnel with care being taken when rotating the insertion of the muscle and accompanying blood vessels. The island of skin is positioned at the recipient site and the skin and muscle sutured into place. Before placing the final sutures, an implant is placed under the muscle to reconstruct the breast mould. The wound is drained with closed suction drains. A nipple–areola reconstruction may be undertaken at this time using groin, auricular or tissue from the unaffected nipple.

If a **transrectus abdominis** flap is performed, the patient is positioned slightly flexed in a supine position. The recipient breast site is prepared. An elliptical incision in made in the lower abdomen and the transverse rectus abdominis muscle is dissected and tunnelled with its pedicle subcutaneously to the midline to the operation site. The flap is rotated so the thickest portion is inferior and lateral, and the thinnest portion is superior and medial. The flap is trimmed into shape and sutured into position. The thickness of this flap usually precludes the necessity of an implant. The opposite breast may need to be altered with a reduction mammoplasty to retain symmetry. A nipple–areola reconstruction may be undertaken at this time using groin, auricular or tissue from the unaffected nipple.

Rhytidectomy (facelift)

A rhytidectomy is the removal of excess skin of the face and neck regions and the tightening of underlying support structures. The procedure is performed to improve the appearance of the patient by removing skin around the face and neck that has become loose and redundant usually as the result of the ageing process.

The patient is placed in a supine position and the face and hair bordering the face is prepared with an aqueous antimicrobial solution. The incision lines are made in the hair or close to the hairline and where possible follow the natural folds of the skin. Bilateral incision lines are made from the temporal scalp, in front of the ear in a natural skin wrinkle line, around the earlobe, onto the posterior surface of the ear and into the occipital scalp. Large flaps of skin and subcutaneous tissue are elevated from the face and upper third of the neck. The superficial muscular aponeurotic system and platysma are tightened, trimmed, and sutured behind and above the ears.[1] Sutures are placed in the musculofacial tissues and tension is placed on the flap pulling the flap superiorly and posteriorly. The excess fat is trimmed and the neck contoured either by removing excess fatty tissue or by suctioning. The skin edges are excised of excess skin and the incisions are closed with fine sutures.

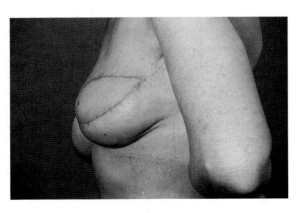

Fig. 8.55 Breast reconstruction

Drains may be inserted before closure. A light pressure dressing is applied.

Reduction of fractured zygoma

Reduction of a fractured zygoma is the anatomical realignment of the zygoma. The zygoma is elevated to relieve a depression in the cheek on the affected side and to facilitate the ability to open and close the mouth properly. The fractures can be at the zygomatic arch or where the zygoma joins the frontal, temporal and maxillary bones at the suture lines (trimalar fracture). The zygomatic arch fracture is usually treated by closed reduction whereas the trimalar fractures are most often corrected by an open reduction with internal fixation.

The patient is placed in a supine position and the skin is prepared with an aqueous antimicrobial solution. The facial area is draped with a head drape. For the closed reduction, a small incision is made in the hairline at the temple on the affected side. A malar elevator or elevator of choice is inserted and the fractured bone elevated. The incision site is closed.

For the open reduction of the trimalar fracture, incisions are made in the orbital rim in the eyebrow line and lower eyelid above the fracture sites. The depressed bone is elevated with an elevator. Holes are drilled in the fractured bone on each side of the fractured bone and wires are placed through the holes and twisted down to reduce the fracture. Alternatively a small plate may be placed across the fracture lines and fixated with screws. It is usually sufficient to fixate only two of the three fractures. The incision sites are closed.

OPHTHALMOLOGICAL SURGERY

Ophthalmological surgery involves procedures aimed at restoring vision lost through disease, injury or congenital defects. These procedures are performed on the external and internal structures of the eye. These structures consist of the bony orbit, the eyelids and eyelashes, the conjunctiva and lacrimal apparatus, the layers of the eyeball, the muscles of the eye, the nerve and blood supply, and the refractive apparatus.

The **bony orbit** consists of seven bones formed posteriorly around the vital structures of the eye to form a protective cavity: the maxilla, palatine, frontal, sphenoidal, zygomatic, ethmoid and lacrimal. The periosteum of the orbital walls is continuous with the dura mater.

Anteriorly, the **eyelids** and **eyelashes** protect the eye. The lids consist of two musculofibrous folds in front of each orbit with the upper lid being larger and more mobile than the lower eyelid. The eyelid is closed by the orbicular muscle of the eye and opened by the levator muscle from above and relaxation of the orbicular muscle. The free margins of the lid have two or three rows of hairs called eyelashes. The eyelids distribute secretions that keep the cornea moist and wash away small foreign particles.

The **conjunctiva** is a thin, transparent membrane that lines the back surface of the eyelids (palpebral) and the front surface of the eyeball (bulbar). The conjunctiva forms a sac that opens anteriorly. The palpebral part contains the openings of the lacrimal ducts that establish a passageway between the conjunctival sac and the inferior meatus of the nose. The bulbar part is transparent, allowing the sclera or white of the eye to show through. The **lacrimal apparatus** consists of the lacrimal gland that produces tears and secretes them through a series of ducts onto the surface of the eyeball where they bathe the conjunctival sac. The tears continue inwards to the puncta where they are collected by the lacrimal ducts and pass into the lacrimal sac and finally into the nasal duct via the nasolacrimal duct.

The **globe (eyeball)** is supported within the orbit on a cushion of fat and fascia and is comprised of three layers surrounding a fluid-filled centre. The fluid contents are aqueous humour in front of the lens and vitreous humour in the posterior section of the eye.

The **external layer** is the corneal–scleral fibrous protective layer comprised of the transparent avascular anterior section called the cornea, and the posterior opaque part called the sclera. The epithelial layer of the cornea consists of five or six constantly renewing cell layers and nerve endings that account for corneal sensitivity. The Bowman's layer is comprised of connective tissue that forms a barrier to trauma and infection. Scarring is left if this layer is damaged as it will not regenerate. The inner endothelial cell layer will also not regenerate and is responsible for the correct amount of dehydration that will keep the cornea clear. Damage to this layer causes corneal oedema and loss of transparency.[1] The sclera is pierced by the ciliary arteries and nerves and posteriorly by the optic nerve. It also receives the tendons of the muscles of the eyeball.

The **middle layer** of the eye comprises the choroid, ciliary body and iris. The iris is in front of the lens and is attached to the ciliary body. The centre forms an aperture known as the pupil that dilates and contracts according to the action of the iris. The iris divides the chamber between the cornea and the lens into the anterior and posterior chambers, which are filled with aqueous humour. The amount of light that enters the eye is regulated by the action of the smooth muscle fibres of the iris. As more light strikes the eye, the sphincter action constricts the pupil. The vascular choroid is the main source of nourishment of the receptor cell and pigment epithelial layer of the retina. The ciliary body contains muscle tissue that aids in accommodation and neuroepithelium that is continuous with the retina and is responsible for secretion of aqueous humour.[1]

The **inner layer** is the retina that is comprised of a thin transparent membrane extending from the ora serrata to the optic disk. The function of this network of nerve cells and fibres is to receive images of external objects and transfer the impression via the optic nerve to the occipital lobe of the cerebrum. The ten

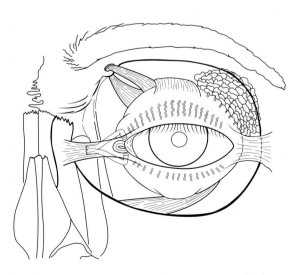

Fig. 8.56 Anatomy of the eye

Perioperative care of adults

layers of the retina consist of photoreceptor cells (rods and cones), sensory neurons and an epithelial layer that transfers nourishment and oxygen from the choroid.

The **refractive apparatus** consists of the cornea, the aqueous humour, the lens and the vitreous body. The cornea has the greatest refractive power and changes to the curvature of the cornea change its refractive power. The lens is biconvex and can expand and contract by means of the zonular fibres. The crystalline lens cells compress and harden with age and the lens loses its elasticity. The vitreous body is a transparent gelatinous mass that fills four-fifths of the eyeball and is adherent to the retina at the vitreous base. The light waves enter the eye perpendicularly and obliquely and for clear vision the oblique waves must converge and come to focus with the central waves on the retina. The refractory devices of the cornea, aqueous humour, lens and vitreous refract the light waves so that the rays strike the macular area.[1]

The **muscles of the eye** are divided into two groups: intrinsic (inside the eyeball) and extrinsic (attached to the bone and muscle). The intrinsic muscles include the iris and ciliary bodies. There are six striated extrinsic muscles that are inserted into the sclera by tendons: these include four rectus muscles and two oblique muscles. These muscles are responsible for moving the eyeball around various axes, which allows binocular focus to occur.

The **sensory nerves** associated with the eye are the optic nerve, which carries visual impulses received by the rods and cones in the retina to the brain, and the ophthalmic nerve (branch of the fifth cranial nerve), which carries the impulses of pain, touch and temperature from the eye and surrounding areas.

There are three nerves carrying **motor** fibres to the muscles of the eyeball.

- Oculomotor: supplies voluntary and involuntary motor fibres to all rectus muscles except the lateral rectus muscle.
- Trochlear: innervates the superior oblique muscle.
- Abducens: innervates the lateral rectus muscle.

The central retinal artery and vein travel through the optic nerve and provide circulation for the inner retina. The main arterial supply to the orbit and globe is the ophthalmic artery, which is a branch of the internal carotid artery.

Perioperative nursing considerations

The population requiring interventions for ophthalmological procedures will include both children and adults with only adults being discussed here. Ophthalmological patients are often admitted only for the day and their care and planning will include admission and discharge information. An assessment should be undertaken of their home environment and self-care needs to plan for their education and discharge requirements. For patients undergoing ophthalmological surgery, a nursing assessment should involve the routine questions to obtain an accurate nursing and medical history. Conditions that have resulted in visual loss and symptoms resulting from this loss should be documented and noted by the perioperative nurse. These may include medical problems such as diabetes, eye disease, cardiovascular disease, hypertension, or drug allergy. Provision will need to be made to accommodate any physiological impairment during the perioperative stages.

There are other possible nursing considerations.

- Seeking the patient's cooperation and confidence by speaking softly and distinctly, and endeavouring to keep the patient quiet and relaxed by staying close and establishing contact by touch during the procedure if under monitored local anaesthetic.
- Observation of general physical appearance to assess skin integrity especially in the elderly.
- Permission given for the patient to wear spectacles for as long as possible if required.
- Communicate with the patient by touching their arm to get their attention or approaching them from the unaffected side to avoid startling them.
- The provision of tissues to wipe any drops or secretions from the eye.
- Note any previous problems with anaesthesia.
- Ensuring any X-rays, MRI scans, CAT scans and any other test results are present in the theatre for review.
- Observation of any limitations in mobility.
- Identification of the correct eye for surgery.
- Advise the patient to avoid activities that increase intraocular pressure postsurgery.
- Ensure methods of keeping the patient warm are available.
- Advise the patient that they may have their eyelashes trimmed.

SURGICAL INTERVENTIONS

Surgery of the eye is performed to restore function and vision to the eyeball and surrounding structures. The most common surgical procedures performed on the eye are a cataract extraction and insertion of an intraocular lens, repair of a retinal detachment or surgery for strabismus. Most intra- and some extraocular procedures are performed with the aid of the operating microscope.

The patient is placed in a supine position for most ophthalmological surgery with the arm on the unaffected side on an armboard if required and the head positioned in a securing headrest. The eyelid and surrounding area is prepared with the appropriate antimicrobial solution with care being taken to prevent solution from entering the eye. Special armrests either on the surgeon's chair or as part of the patient's headrest will need to be covered with sterile covers. Lint-free drapes should be used for ophthalmic surgery.

Cataract extraction and insertion of intraocular lens

Cataract extraction is performed to remove an opaque ocular lens. Blurred vision may be the result of injury causing dislocation of the lens, a congenital defect or opacification caused by ageing, disease or certain medications. Cataracts can vary in density, size and location and are one of the most common causes of gradual, painless loss of vision.

There are three main types of cataract extraction procedures.

- Intracapsular: cataract is removed while still within its capsule.
- Extracapsular: anterior portion of the capsule is removed; the lens cortex and nucleus is expressed from the eye leaving behind the posterior capsule.
- Phacoemulsification: contents of the lens capsule are fragmented with ultrasonic energy as the lens material is irrigated and aspirated.

Intracapsular cataract extraction

A lid speculum is placed in the eye to hold the lids apart. A traction suture is placed through the superior rectus muscle to hold the eye in place and to

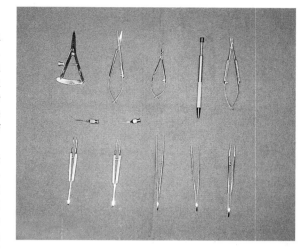

Fig. 8.57 Eye instruments

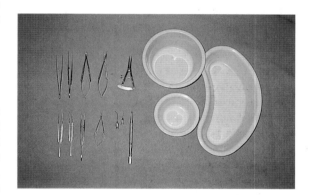

Fig. 8.58 Ophthalmological instruments

control the rotation of the globe. A small bulldog or mosquito forceps may be placed on the ends of the suture. An incision is made into the conjunctiva and bleeding points are cauterised by means of bipolar diathermy forceps or eraser diathermy. A diamond knife is used to enter through the limbus and into the anterior chamber and an iridotomy is performed. Sutures may be applied at the edges of the incision at this stage. An enzymatic solution is injected through the iridotomy to dissolve the fibres suspending the lens. A cryoextractor is applied to the lens and the lens is withdrawn from the eye. If an intraocular lens implant is to be used, it will be inserted following the extraction of the lens from the eye. The prosthesis may be sutured to the iris or held in place by its shape depending on the type of prosthesis. The limbic incision is closed with the anterior chamber being irrigated with a balanced salt solution to restore its shape just before tying of the last suture. The suture line is checked for leakage. The pupil may be constricted with the use of acetylcholine drops (Miochol) once the lens has been inserted. The rectus muscle suture is cut and the conjunctival flap reapproximated and sutured into position. Subconjunctival antibiotic injections may be used to prevent inflammation and infection. Some surgeons may use antibiotic ointment topically for the same purpose. The eye is dressed with an eye pad and eye shield, which are secured with tape.

Extracapsular cataract extraction

This procedure is the same as for an intracapsular cataract extraction up to removal of the lens. A lid speculum is placed in the eye to hold the lids apart. A traction suture is placed through the superior rectus muscle to hold the eye in place and to control the rotation of the globe. A small bulldog or mosquito forceps may be placed on the ends of the suture. An incision is made into the conjunctiva and bleeding points are cauterised by means of bipolar diathermy forceps or eraser diathermy. A diamond knife is used to enter through the limbus and into the anterior chamber. Healon (or other viscoelastic) is used to fill the anterior chamber to prevent damage to the endothelial layer of the cornea. A cystotome is used to perforate the anterior lens capsule and an anterior capsulotomy is performed. The capsule fragment is removed with the Kelman McPherson forceps. The limbic incision is extended with the diamond knife or scissors. Sutures may be applied at the edges of the incision at this stage. The lens nucleus is expressed from the eye with the aid of a lens hook and the remnants of the anterior cortex are removed with an irrigation/aspiration cannula system (Simcoe or McIntyre). The lens to be inserted is checked for correct size and received onto the sterile set-up where it is rinsed with the balanced salt solution. The lens is then inserted into the posterior chamber lens capsule and positioned correctly. The anterior chamber is irrigated and aspirated to remove any viscoelastic solution. The limbic incision is closed with fine sutures with the anterior chamber being inflated with

balanced salt solution just before tying of the last suture. The pupil may be constricted with the use of acetylcholine drops (Miochol) once the lens has been inserted. The rectus muscle suture is cut and the conjunctival flap reapproximated and sutured into position. Subconjunctival antibiotic injections may be used to prevent inflammation and infection. Some surgeons may use antibiotic ointment topically for the same purpose. The eye is dressed with an eye pad and eye shield, which are secured with tape (P. Cummings, Ophthalmological Clinical Nurse, Princess Alexandra Hospital, Brisbane, personal communication, 2001).

Phacoemulsification

This procedure has the benefit of a smaller incision than the more traditional extracapsular cataract extraction. A lid speculum is placed in the eye to hold the lids apart. A traction suture is placed through the superior rectus muscle to hold the eye in place and to control the rotation of the globe. A small bulldog or mosquito forceps may be placed on the ends of the suture. A small incision is made into the eye with a diamond knife. A viscoelastic solution may be inserted before using a keratome blade to widen the incision. The lens capsule is opened with a cystotome and forceps are used to tear a small hole in the capsule. A hydrodissection cannula attached to a 2ml syringe of balanced salt solution is used to separate the lens nucleus from the cortex. The phacoemulsification ('phaco') handpiece is checked and primed ready for use and then inserted into the eye. After the lens nucleus is emulsified and removed, the lens cortex is removed with the irrigation/aspiration handpiece. If an intraocular lens is to be inserted, the incision is extended to accommodate the width of the lens and the procedure for insertion of the lens is the same as for an extracapsular cataract extraction.

Repair of a retinal detachment

A repair of a retinal detachment is the reattachment of the retina. The surgery involves sealing off the area in which the tear or hole is located and may include drainage of subretinal fluid. Common surgical methods may include scleral buckling using episcleral and intrascleral techniques, cryotherapy and diathermy.

Retinal detachment is a separation of the neural retinal layer from the pigmented epithelium layer of the retina.[1] Diseases, tumours, degeneration and trauma are all contributing causes to retinal detachment. Fluid from the vitreous cavity and blood from injury can seep through the retinal tears and separate the retinal components causing that part of the retina to become detached from its nutritional source. This separation results in damage and loss of function of that portion of the retina. The aim of prompt treatment of retinal detachment is to prevent loss of central vision and function by returning the retina to its normal anatomical position.

The conjunctiva is incised to the predetermined length using plain forceps and scissors. The four rectus muscles are captured with silk ties to allow mobilisation of the eyeball. With the indirect ophthalmoscope the abnormality is identified under direct visualisation. Cryotherapy and the Mira diathermy are often used under direct visualisation to cause a sterile inflammatory reaction, which leads to a permanent adhesion between the detached retina and the underlying structure. For the buckling procedure, a groove is made around the equator of the eye with a hockey stick blade to permit insertion of an encircling band. If subretinal fluid is to be drained, a small incision is made through the remaining layer of the sclera down to the choroid. The choroid is punctured to allow the subretinal fluid to drain and the puncture site repaired. The band is sutured onto the sclera with fine looped sutures and the indirect ophthalmoscope is used to check the position of the retina. The conjunctival wound is closed and the eye is dressed.

Surgery for strabismus

Strabismus surgery is the alignment of the visual axes of the eyes by changing the relative strength of muscles. These procedures can be performed by two basic surgical approaches. Strengthening is accomplished by a resection procedure, which is the shortening of the extraocular muscle by removing a portion of the muscle and the reanastomosis of the cut ends. Weakening is accomplished by a recession procedure, which is the lengthening of the extraocular muscle by detaching it from its original insertion and reattaching it more posteriorly on the sclera.[2]

The objective of strabismus surgery is to direct the focus of the two eyes at the same object by aiding the coordination of the muscles of the eyeball.

Resection procedure

A speculum is inserted to keep the lids retracted. An incision is made in the conjunctiva at the limbus and extended back to reveal the attachment of the muscle to be resected. A muscle hook is passed under the muscle to ensure that it is free of adhesions and the distance to be resected measured with a calliper. A muscle clamp is placed over the muscle at the selected distance and the muscle excised. The muscle end is reattached to the muscle stump by placing double armed sutures through each end and carefully pulling the two ends of muscle together whilst tying. Haemostasis is achieved and the conjunctival incision closed. The eye is dressed with a pad and shield.

Recession procedure

A speculum is inserted to keep the lids retracted. An incision is made in the conjunctiva at the limbus and extended back to reveal the attachment of the muscle to be recessed. Sutures are passed through the upper and lower edges of the muscles including the anterior ciliary arteries. The muscle is severed from the globe distal to the sutures. The distance of the desired amount of recession is measured from the original insertion point to the desired reattachment point with a calliper. The muscle is anchored to the globe at this point. The conjunctiva is closed and the eye dressed with a pad and shield (Cummings, personal communication, 2001).

ORTHOPAEDIC SURGERY

Orthopaedic surgery involves procedures that restore and preserve the functions of the musculoskeletal system of the body. This system is comprised of the bones, articulations (joints) and skeletal muscles that provide support and movement to the body.

The skeleton is comprised of 206 bones that form the axial and appendicular framework which supports the soft tissue structures of the body. The axial skeleton is comprised of the bones that form the upright axis of the body and the bones of the middle ear. The bones that articulate with the upright skeleton are the appendages that form the appendicular skeleton. Bone is continuously regenerating and being reabsorbed according to the individual's metabolism and absorption of calcium, vitamin D and phosphorus.[1] Periosteum is the layer of connective tissue that covers all bone. Bones perform the following functions.[2]

- Providing a support framework for the body.
- Providing protection for delicate structures and major organs.
- Acting as a reservoir for calcium deposits.
- Serving as a site for haemopoiesis.
- Providing mobility and movement through muscular attachment.

Bones can be classified according to their primary shape and location:[2]

- long bones of the upper and lower extremities, e.g. femur, humerus;
- short bones of the wrist and ankles, e.g. carpals and tarsals;
- irregular bones in the spinal column and cranium, e.g. vertebrae, mandible;
- round bone found within tendons, e.g. patella; and
- flat bones of the thorax, cranium, pelvis and shoulder, e.g. frontal bone, ribs and scapula.

Cortical bone tissue is hard and dense to provide support, e.g. the hard outer shell of the femur, whereas cancellous bone tissue is soft and spongy and is within the inner section of bone such as the pelvic bone or at the end of long bones. It contains red bone marrow for haemopoiesis. The Haversian system is a network of channels that contain blood vessels and nerves to allow the flow of nutrients and facilitate calcium absorption within the bone.[1]

Joints are articulations where bones join. The three basic joints are classified by the type of material between them (fibrous, cartilaginous, synovial) or according to their range of movement (immovable, slightly movable, freely movable).

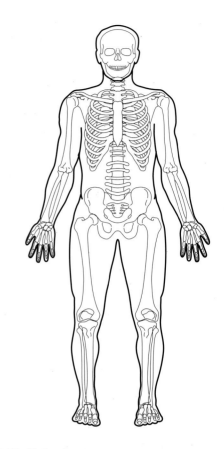

Fig. 8.59 Skeletal system

- **Fibrous** tissue or ligaments connect the immovable joints (synarthrotic), e.g. suture lines of the bones of the skull.
- **Cartilage** connects the slightly movable joints (amphiarthrotic), e.g. symphysis pubis.
- Synovial membrane lines the **synovial** joints and these have one or more ranges of movement, e.g. knee or the hip. Synovial joints can be further divided according to their structure and the kind of movements they permit:[2]
  - **ball and socket**, e.g. hip, shoulder;
  - **hinge**, e.g. knee, elbow;
  - **pivot**, e.g. first and second cervical vertebrae;
  - **ellipsoidal**, e.g. radius and carpal bones;
  - **saddle**, e.g. joints between the metacarpal bone of the thumb and carpal bone; and
  - **gliding**, e.g. most joints of the ankle.

Other structures that also form part of the skeletal system are the bursae, tendons, ligaments and cartilage. Bursae are small connective tissue sacs filled with synovial fluid that reduce friction between movable parts of the joints. Tendons are a group of connective tissue that form the ends of muscles and attach the muscle to bone. They transfer forces to the bone or cartilage to facilitate movement. Ligaments are strong cords of dense white fibrous connective tissue holding the bones together. They stabilise the joint by encircling or holding the ends of bone in place. Cartilage is a layer of tough elastic tissue found mostly at the ends of bones forming a protective coating. It provides a smooth gliding surface for joint movement. It can also be found in other areas such as the nose or ears providing a supporting structure.

The muscles of the skeletal system are masses of tissue composed of bundles of elongated cells capable of contraction and relaxation to produce movement of the bones and joints of the skeleton. These skeletal muscles provide the following functions.

- Maintaining posture by their continued partial contraction of muscles that support the positions of standing, sitting, etc.
- Producing heat by a process known as catabolism. Skeletal muscle cells are highly active and numerous and therefore produce a major share of the total body heat.
- Producing movement of a part of the body or the whole body by the contraction and relaxation of the muscles attached to the bony skeleton.

Perioperative nursing considerations

For patients undergoing orthopaedic surgery, nursing assessment involves the routine questions to obtain an accurate nursing and medical history. Special attention should be given to physical conditions associated with the problems that have brought the patient to surgery. For example, if the patient's admission is the result of road trauma, then there may be other major injuries that need to be considered during positioning. These patients may experience major alterations to their body image as limbs and faces may have been severely damaged. The population requiring interventions for orthopaedic

procedures will include the entire age range. Many patients will be fit and healthy adults undergoing surgery after trauma but will be experiencing anxiety related to their surgical outcome.

Other nursing considerations may be the following.

- Observation of the general physical appearance to assess skin integrity especially in the elderly.
- Note any previous problems with anaesthesia. Drug reactions to local anaesthetic should be noted as these agents may be used extensively during this surgery.
- Ensuring any X-rays, scans, consultations with other surgeons and any other tests are present in the theatre for review.
- Observation for any limitations in mobility especially of the joints in the elderly patient.
- Ensuring availability of the correct operating table and equipment for positioning of the patient to maintain body alignment and provide adequate exposure of the operative area is available.
- Ensuring equipment to keep the patient warm is available as some procedures can be lengthy.
- Checking that equipment and prosthesis for the procedure have been delivered and are sterilised ready for use.
- If power equipment is to be used, ensure that there is enough tool air or cylinder gas to complete the procedure.
- Ensure there are sufficient staff to move the patient as they may be in considerable pain due to the damage to their limbs.
- Check that the correct site is identified for surgery.
- If supervision is required to move the patient, ensure the surgeon is available.
- If intraoperative X-rays need to be taken, ensure the X-ray technician has been booked.

SURGICAL INTERVENTIONS

Orthopaedic surgery is performed to repair or correct deformities in bone and/or soft tissue, repair fractured bone, reconstruct a joint, and to perform diagnostic examinations to determine the extent of damage to a joint.[2] Similar orthopaedic procedures can be performed on the musculoskeletal system throughout the body using different sizes of the same prosthesis, e.g. repairs to a fracture of the carpal or radius using plates and screws. Some of the more common procedures will be described as examples of basic techniques and operative procedures. It should be noted that surgeons in other specialities also perform some procedures performed by orthopaedic surgeons, e.g. hand surgery by plastic and reconstructive surgeons, and spinal surgery by neurosurgeons.

The principles of the aseptic technique should be strictly adhered to in orthopaedic surgery, especially when inserting implants. It is important to allow the antimicrobial skin preparation solution to dry thoroughly before applying the adhesive drapes. Tourniquets should be applied correctly and the time of avascularity recorded. Positioning will depend on the operation to be performed and it is important to prevent further damage to affected limbs or other healthy tissues.

Repairs of fractured bone

Fractures can be treated by several different surgical methods, but first the fracture must be brought into alignment and then stabilised. The method chosen will depend on the type of fracture. Fractures are classified by type, location and direction.

- Closed non-displaced: bone is broken and the ends are still in contact with each other.
- Open compound: bone is broken and communicates with the surface either through the skin or a wound site.
- Comminuted: bone is shattered into several pieces.
- Displaced: bone is misaligned at the fracture site.
- Spiral: fracture line twists around the bone shaft.
- Impacted: one bone fragment is driven into the other.
- Oblique: fracture line crosses the longitudinal axis of the bone shaft at 45°.
- Greenstick: incomplete fracture where one side is broken and the other left bent. Most commonly found in children.
- Pathological: bone is weakened for some pathological reason and stress causes it to fracture.

Fractures are treated to restore anatomical function and re-establish the length, shape and alignment of the fractured bones. This process can be accomplished by four different methods of treatment: closed reduction and stabilisation, closed reduction and external fixation, closed reduction and internal fixation, and open reduction and internal fixation.

Closed reduction

A closed reduction is the manual manipulation of the fractured bone into position without incising the skin. The alignment is confirmed with an X-ray film or an image intensifier and the affected limb is immobilised in a cast. Closed reduction is usually carried out for closed non-displaced fractures. This treatment decreases the opportunity for infection and reduces the length of hospital stay.

Closed reduction and external fixation

A closed reduction of the fracture is performed and an external fixation system is inserted into the bone percutaneously to maintain alignment. The external fixation system attached to the pins provides rigid fixation and reduction with the ability to manage severe soft tissue wounds. This system is indicated when there are severe open fractures usually with bony loss, infected joints, highly comminuted closed fractures, infected non-union of fractures, length deficits, and when other procedures such as grafts and flaps need to be performed.

The fracture is manually reduced and alignment is confirmed with an X-ray film. Small incisions are made in the skin and pins are drilled into the bone using a drill sleeve to protect the surrounding soft tissue. At this stage, a simple traction apparatus may be applied. If an external fixation frame is to be applied, after the pins have been inserted into the bone, universal clamps will be slipped over the pins and connected with longitudinal supporting devices (rods). The frame is adjusted and tightened with the appropriate wrenches and the pin sites dressed. The more sophisticated systems are radio-opaque and can utilise the principles of tension–stress and distraction to correct bone defects and limb length discrepancies (e.g. Ilizarov external fixation system).

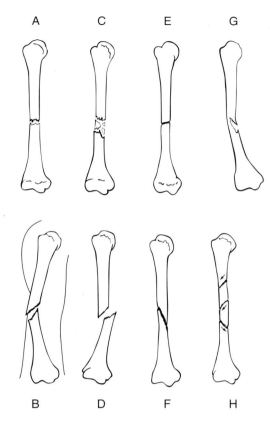

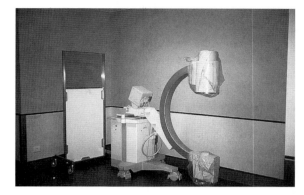

Fig. 8.61 Image intensifier

Fig. 8.60 Fracture sites: A, closed, non-displaced; B, open compound; C, comminuted; D, displaced; E, impacted; F, oblique; G, greenstick; H, spiral

Closed reduction and internal fixation

Closed reduction and internal fixation is the manual reduction of the fracture and the percutaneous insertion of pins, intramedullary nails or rods. The advantage of the method is the lower risk of infection and absence of additional soft tissue and vascular damage. The prosthesis inserted must be relative to the size of the bone and fracture site, e.g. Kirschner wire for the distal phalanx and nails for large bones. For large bones, a small incision is made to insert the nails or rods, but it is considerably smaller than for an open reduction. The guide rod is placed across the fracture to maintain the alignment, the cancellous bone may or may not be reamed, and a nail or rod driven through the medulla and across the fracture site to stabilise the fracture. The wound is closed and dressed.

Open reduction and internal fixation

An open reduction and internal fixation is the realignment and fixation of a fracture necessitating visualisation of the fracture site via an operative incision. The procedure is performed when satisfactory reduction of a fracture cannot be obtained or maintained with closed methods. The procedure described uses a dynamic compression plate and screws to stabilise the fracture.

An incision is made over the fracture site and the surrounding periosteum may need to be carefully cleaned away from the fracture with an elevator. The fracture is reduced and the fragments reapproximated utilising bone reduction and grasping forceps. The fracture site is assessed for the size of plate to be used. A dynamic compression plate is selected and placed with the correct number of holes above and below the fracture. A concentric hole is drilled through one of the screw holes on the plate to the opposite cortex. The depth of the hole is gauged and the selected size screw inserted, ensuring purchase of the opposite cortex. A second screw is inserted on the opposite fragment in the neutral position. An eccentric (loading) hole is drilled on either side of the fracture to the opposite cortex. The hole is gauged, tapped and the screw inserted compressing the fracture site. After this screw is tightened down, the other screws are loosened slightly. The remaining screws are inserted following the same procedure. The wound is irrigated and closed. A dressing is applied and the limb supported in an appropriate device.

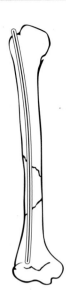

Fig. 8.62 Intramedullary rod fixation

Reconstruction of joints

An arthroplasty of the joint is performed to restore motion of the joint and function to the muscles and ligaments.[1] The surgical procedure is indicated in patients with a disabling arthritic joint, degenerative diseases or avascular necrosis following a failed reconstruction, infection in the joint, or a fractured neck of femur. Joint replacements may be performed on most joints of the body including the hip, knee, shoulder, elbow, wrist, ankle, metatarsal and metacarpal (using Silastic™ implants). Joint revision may be necessary due to infection, dislocation, fracture, wear and tear on the prosthesis or when the primary replacement was performed at an early age. Allograft bone may be used to replace bony loss. The work practices of the operating staff and environment within the operating room may play a role in the success or failure of total joint implantation. The outcome of infection after receiving an implant in these patients can be catastrophic with loss of mobility and destruction of their lifestyle. The risk of airborne and contact contamination should be minimised by strict adherence to aseptic technique, draping technique, traffic control and proper operating room attire. Prophylactic antibiotics are usually administered before, during and after surgery.

Total hip replacement

A total hip replacement is the substitution of the femoral head and acetabulum with a prosthesis that may or may not be fixed using bone cement. This surgical procedure is performed for patients with hip pain due to degenerative joint disease or rheumatoid arthritis. Many prostheses are available and the procedure can be cemented, non-cemented or be a combination (hybrid) where the femoral shaft is cemented and the acetabular cup is not. Prostheses are made from various substances such as metal, porous metal, ceramic, polyethylene or varying combinations. No one prosthesis is suitable for every patient. Therefore, a variety of types, designs and insertion procedures are available and dependent on the pathophysiological needs of the patient.

The patient is placed in the lateral position with side plates supporting the torso. The arms are placed in a flexed position on arm supports. The unaffected leg is extended with the affected leg flexed over it with a pillow placed between the legs. The patient's skin is prepared with an antimicrobial solution from mid-chest to the foot and to the bedline laterally including the groin. The operative area is defined by sterile, lint-free drapes.

■ A longitudinal incision is made proximal to the greater trochanter and distal along the proximal femoral shaft. The hip joint capsule is exposed by dissection through the muscle, identifying the nerves and vessels, and tagging the rotators with a suture before release.

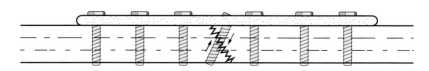

Fig. 8.63 Dynamic compression plate application

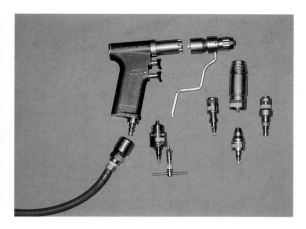

Fig. 8.64 Orthopaedic drill

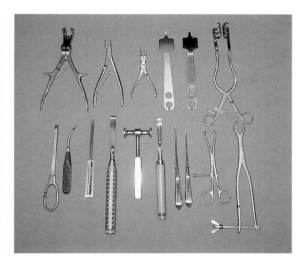

Fig. 8.65 A range of Orthopaedic instruments

- A capsulotomy is performed to release the femoral head and after manipulating the leg into internal rotation; the femoral head is dislocated and exposed.
- The femoral head is cut with a saw (osteotomy) at a level determined by the type of implant to be used. At this stage, either the acetabular or femoral procedure will be performed depending on the type of prosthesis used.
- The acetabulum is cleared of osteophytes, cysts and cartilage with large curettes, osteotomes or a nibbler. The acetabulum is reamed with acetabu-

lar reamers and anchor holes are drilled in the floor of the acetabulum if bone cement is to be used. An acetabular component is trialled.

- A high-viscosity cement (with or without antibiotics) is prepared and placed into the acetabular cavity and pressurised to remove air. The acetabular shell component is positioned and held motionless with the appropriate equipment until the cement polymerises. Excess cement is removed from around the edge of the component.
- The femoral canal is opened using a box chisel or reamer and reamed using increasing sizes in broaches until the cortical bone is reached. A femoral component is trialled.
- The component is removed and the canal cleaned with hydrogen peroxide to remove blood and debris. A femoral canal cement plug is inserted into the femoral canal to prevent cement reaching the bottom of the canal and to facilitate easy removal if necessary.
- A prepared low-viscosity cement is injected into the canal with a cement gun and pressurised. The femoral prosthetic component is inserted, excess cement is removed and the cement allowed to harden.
- A trial head is placed on the femoral component and the hip is reduced. The joint is taken through a range of motions in flexion, extension and rotation to test for dislocation. The leg length is assessed. The appropriately sized prosthetic head is positioned and the hip reduced.
- The wound is sutured in layers with suction drains inserted. The skin is approximated with skin clips and the wound dressed. The patient will be positioned with an abduction pillow between their legs postoperatively. **Postoperatively, patient positioning and teaching are extremely important aspects of care as dislocation of the femur is a serious complication** (A. Hamilton, Orthopaedic Clinical Nurse, Princess Alexandra Hospital, Brisbane, personal communication, 2001).

Total knee replacement

A total knee replacement is the surgical procedure to replace the worn articular surfaces of the knee joint by prosthesis. This procedure is indicated for severe destruction of the knee joint due to degenerative, rheumatoid or traumatic arthritis. Only one articular surface may be replaced by prosthesis, but more commonly the total surface requires replacement.

The patient is placed in a supine position with a tourniquet applied to the upper thigh. The skin is prepared with an antimicrobial solution from the lower border of the tourniquet cuff for the entire length of the leg, including the foot. The leg is draped with lint-free drapes to expose the appropriate operative site with the leg below the knee encased in an impervious stockinette to facilitate ease of movement.

- A longitudinal incision is made over the knee. The capsule is entered and inspected and any osteophytes are removed. The knee is flexed, the infrapatellar fat pad is excised and the patella everted.
- The tibial jig is attached to the tibia to correct deficiency in the tibial plateau and to obtain alignment. The tibial cut is performed to create a flat surface and the tibial component is sized.
- A central hole is drilled in the distal femur and a series of anterior cutting blocks are attached and assembled. The femoral component size is determined. With correct alignment being maintained, the final guided oblique corner cuts are completed and the prosthesis trialled.
- Depending on the type of prosthesis used, a central hole is made in the tibia for insertion of a peg. The peg and tibial base plate are trialled.
- The patella is measured and cut to correspond with the femoral component. A trial is attached.
- With all the trial components in place, the knee is assessed for its range of movement and stability.
- The trial components are removed and the joint surfaces are cleaned with a pulsatile lavage. The cement is mixed and applied to the bone surfaces and the tibial, femoral and patella prostheses are attached. Excess bone cement is removed and the edges cleaned. The joint is reduced and a final inspection and range of motion are performed.
- The wound is closed in layers and suction drains are inserted. The skin is approximated with skin clips and a dressing applied. Depending on the surgeon preference, a splint may be applied to provide additional support (Hamilton, personal communication, 2001).

Arthroscopy of a joint

Arthroscopic surgery may be performed on any joint and can be diagnostic or operative depending on the condition of the patient. Diagnostic arthroscopy is indicated for patients whose condition cannot be determined by other examinations or studies (X-ray or history). An operative arthroscopy is performed when an intra-articular abnormality or damage from injury is known. Indications for arthroscopic surgery include synovial biopsies, removal of torn meniscus and removal of loose bodies.

Arthroscopy of the knee

An arthroscopy of the knee is the direct visualisation of the knee joint using an arthroscope. The procedure is indicated for diagnostic viewing, synovial biopsies, removal of loose bodies, shaving of the meniscus, synovectomy, partial meniscectomy, meniscus repair and anterior cruciate ligament reconstruction.[1]

The patient is placed in a supine position and the end of the operating table can be flexed by 90° (depends on the surgeon's preference). A tourniquet is applied and the leg prepared with an antimicrobial solution. An arthroscopic drape is placed that allows a full range of motion of the leg and evacuation of the irrigating solution.

An irrigating trocar and cannula are placed after a small stab incision is made into the suprapatellar pouch. The joint is distended with the appropriate irrigating solution (normal saline). Further stab incisions are made either anterolaterally or medially to facilitate the insertion of an additional trocar and cannula through the capsule. The sharp trocar is removed after the capsule is breached and using a blunt trocar the cannula is progressed further. The arthroscope (videoscope) is inserted and the light source, camera, irrigation and drainage tubing connected. The knee contents are visually examined. If a procedure is undertaken, the operative instrument is introduced into the joint under direct visualisation and the procedure completed. Special instrumentation (chrondrotome) may be used to remove damaged meniscal tissue. Following completion of the examination/procedure, the irrigating solution is allowed to drain from the knee and the stab wounds closed and dressed (Hamilton, personal communication, 2001).

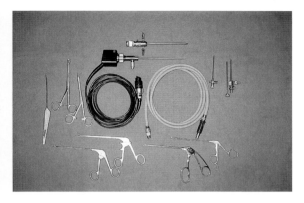

Fig. 8.66 Arthroscopic instruments

PERIOPERATIVE CARE OF THE ELDERLY PATIENT

EFFECTS OF SURGERY ON THE ELDERLY

People aged 65 years and over are the fastest growing segment of the population with an increased life expectancy, and those aged 85 years and older represent the fastest growing portion of this elderly population. It is therefore to be expected that surgery will be performed more frequently on the elderly population as they experience more chronic diseases and disorders that require hospitalisation than younger people do. Age alone is not a contraindication to surgery,[1] but the decision to perform surgery is an evaluation by the surgeon more of the risk of not operating than evaluating the comparative risks seen in a younger patient. The surgeon would need to evaluate the life expectancy of the patient with the natural course of the disease, whether the operation will result in the patient maintaining an independent lifestyle and whether the patient is motivated to do all that is necessary to get well. The surgeon would also need to evaluate whether non-operative management may be preferable to the surgical option. Care of the elderly patient during surgery requires attention to their special requirements that result from the ageing processes. The most desirable outcome is to maintain their self-care, not to impair any of their abilities and to prevent any postoperative complications.

To maintain this optimal patient functioning becomes the primary objective in the healthcare management of the elderly surgical patient. An assessment of the physical and mental functions become important indicators of the elderly patient's health and quality of life and highlight any chronic conditions. To the elderly patient, the effects of surgery-related events can be significant. These events may include the anaesthetic, surgery, medications, pain and immobility. The perioperative nurse through an accurate assessment and planned interventions can contribute to the maintenance of the elderly patient's functioning.

Perioperative nursing assessment

The nurse conducts a physical assessment to determine the present physiological functioning of the patient. This assessment provides baseline cardiovascular, respiratory, nervous, gastrointestinal, renal, musculoskeletal, fluid balance, nutritional and mobility statuses. These baseline data is used to plan patient care during the perioperative stages and to identify intra- and postoperative changes to the health status of the elderly surgical patient.

Changes in the physiological functioning of the elderly patient may alter from one person to the next, but in general, the elderly patient can expect changes in the following.

Cardiovascular system

An increased risk of cardiovascular disease may lead to a decreased cardiac output and limited reserves and a decreased ability of the cardiovascular system to tolerate stressors placed on the heart. This disease process also results in a decreased tissue perfusion of other organs such as the kidney and liver.

Respiratory system

Decreased lung capacity results when degenerative changes in thoracic expansion and lung elasticity, reduced alveolar surface, weakening of the respiratory muscles and calcification of the costal cartilages occur.[4] A combination of these changes makes the postoperative patient more susceptible to respiratory infection.

Nervous system

A decrease in neuron numbers causes elderly patients to experience alterations in cognitive functioning and a decrease in some organ systems' ability to transfer reliable messages to the brain. Patients who experience cerebral arteriosclerosis and atherosclerosis may exhibit decreased blood flow and nervous system deficits of irritability, visual motor deficits, sensory losses, memory losses,[1] and losses in the tactile senses of heat and pain perception.

Gastrointestinal system

A decrease in secretion of salivary and digestive glands and a decrease in peristalsis and reduction of gastric motility cause a delay in stomach emptying. The absorption of drugs is affected by this delayed gastric emptying, a reduction of blood flow to the abdominal viscera and hydrochloric acid. Alterations in the total body water and plasma volume, a lean body mass and an increase in the body fat percentage are important factors for consideration when prescribing anaesthetic and postoperative drugs.

Renal system

Renal and hepatic function decreases with age and because of the decreased blood flow to the kidneys and liver, elimination of drugs through the liver and kidneys is affected. An accumulative adverse effect of these drugs is of important consideration during the perioperative period. A decreased ability to conserve sodium can lead to disorientation and confusion, especially in the immediate postoperative period, and therefore fluid balance should be closely monitored. A decrease in the elasticity and tone in the ureters, bladder and urethra can lead to incomplete emptying of the bladder, and men may also experience difficulty in voiding and retention if benign prostatic hypertrophy is present.

Musculoskeletal system

Significant changes to the elderly person's skeleton is affected by arthritic and osteoporotic processes. Joints may be distorted and lose the ability to be flexible, and the vertebrae and hips are susceptible to fractures. Loss of functioning in the temporomandibular joint results in difficulty in intubation, poor fitting of dentures and may lead to poor nutritional status of the patient. Poor abduction and adduction of limbs will make positioning difficult.

Sensory changes

The elderly patient will experience changes to sight, hearing, temperature perception and understanding. It is important that the patient can see and hear explanations that are given and that they are not considered senile because they cannot understand because of these reasons.

Integumentary system

The skin of the elderly patient loses elasticity and subcutaneous fat and is therefore more prone to shearing forces and pressure injury. The skin becomes thin, fragile and the small vessels rupture easily leading to bruising. The loss of subcutaneous fat is one of the contributing factors that alters the thermoregulation ability of the older person; the other is the decreased vascularity of the skin. A good blood supply is necessary to provide the skin with nutrition that promotes wound healing and the capacity for body heat regulation.

Perioperative nursing considerations

During the preoperative visit by the nurse, information can be assembled that will aid in the preparation of the operating environment for the safe care of the elderly patient.

It is important during this interview that the nurse is aware the elderly patient may be experiencing some stressors that may affect her/his replies to the questions asked.

- The patient may be confused about time and place resultant from a slow dementia that has remained undiagnosed at home. These changes of memory loss, problem-solving and information processing can be hidden when the patient has performed the necessary tasks in an environment that is routine, stable and familiar.[5] It needs to be assessed whether this patient can perform additional tasks resulting from surgery (e.g. physiotherapy) in this same environment or whether assistance is required.
- The patient may be experiencing feelings of tension and anxiety about the forthcoming surgery and a potential threat to their self-esteem and independence. Many patients feel their independence is removed when in hospital and the

elderly may see this episode as a real threat to their future independence from relatives and their placement in a nursing facility. This occurs even when the assistance may only be for a short period.

- The preoperative interview should be conducted in a quiet, relaxed environment where there are no distractions. The patient should be allowed to respond to each question independently without prompting from other family members unless absolutely necessary. This will maintain the elderly patient's dignity, independence and control.[1]

- A deterioration in hearing and vision can lead to a misunderstanding of questions asked and therefore inappropriate answers may be given. The nurse must ensure that the elderly patient can hear explanations and see drawings of procedures so that a full understanding of the surgical episode can be obtained. It is also very important that the patient can understand and see the consent form before being asked to sign the form.

- The skin of the elderly patient is often frail and papery and will not withstand shearing forces, pressure or adhesive tapes. An assessment of the condition of the skin allows the perioperative nurse to provide appropriate cushioning, tapes and equipment to allow safe movement onto the operating table. During positioning and skin preparation of the patient, the skin can be examined for signs of injury, particularly over bony prominences and under the electrosurgical dispersive pad. Wet linen should be removed from under the patient postoperatively to prevent skin injury.

- An assessment of the patient's mobility will provide information on the ability of the patient to be placed in the appropriate position for the surgical procedure. The position may need to be modified to accommodate limbs and a spine that no longer has the flexibility to straighten or bend.

- Consent to an operation is important for all patients but especially for the elderly as they wish to make an informed decision about whether the surgery will improve or at least not worsen their existing quality of life. It may be that an elderly patient will refuse surgery if they fear it will not improve their life and healthcare workers must respect this request.

- An assessment of any medications or allergies to solutions used will aid the perioperative nurse to act as an advocate for the patient to ensure incorrect medications are not administered. This assessment should be combined with an assessment for nutritional and dehydration status so accurate quantities of drugs can be administered safely.

- As the elderly patient often has altered responses to pain and temperature, the preoperative assessment can indicate the additional need for warming devices during the surgery.

- Strict adherence to the aseptic technique is essential as the elderly patient has increased susceptibility to poor wound healing.

- The maintenance of an accurate fluid balance account must be maintained by recording all intravenous fluids administered intraoperatively, suction bottle contents, sponges, raytec and urinary drainage bag contents.

Surgical procedures performed on the elderly have as an additional risk the deficits caused by the ageing processes. Procedures performed in the thoracic region have the added risks of poorer air entry and coughing reflexes. Hip and knee surgery is complicated by poorer mobility but is dependent on the condition of the patient preoperatively. No procedure is strictly for the elderly patient as differing types are performed on all ages. With thorough preparation of the perioperative environment, good education of the patient, careful handling of the patient's tissues, and skilful assessment by the anaesthetist and surgeon, surgery for the elderly patient should be uncomplicated and achieve a successful outcome.

References

1. Meeker RH, Rothrock JC. *Alexander's Care of the Patient in Surgery*, 11th edn. St Louis: Mosby, 1995.
2. Fairchild SS. *Perioperative Nursing: Principles and Practice*, 2nd edn. Boston: Little, Brown, 1996.
3. Seifert PC. *Cardiac Surgery*. St Louis: Mosby, 1994.
4. Curry M. Perioperative nursing care of the elderly patient: a case study. *ACORN J* 1994; 7: 23–26.
5. Lusis SA. The challenges of nursing elderly surgical patients. *AORN J* 1996; 64: 954–962.

Perioperative care of children

4

9 | Psychosocial care of children in the perioperative area

Linda Shields and Lee-Anne Waterman

EFFECT OF HOSPITALISATION ON CHILDREN

Linda Shields

In all discussions about children in this book, the word 'parent' is taken to mean the child's natural parent, step-parent, legal guardian or carer.

There has been some research into the emotional effect of surgery and operative procedures on children, and the effect of hospitalisation has been studied extensively. Over the years, admission to hospital has been portrayed as a positive, growth-promoting experience for children.[1] Blom[2] in 1958 inferred that tonsillectomy was emotionally good for children. In 1973, hospitalisation was described as a growth experience.[3] As late as 1992, Lansdown suggested that children could gain psychologically from a hospital admission.[4] Strachan[5] investigated psychological trauma encountered by children aged 3–7 years, and their parents, before admission for routine ear, nose and throat (ENT) surgery and highlighted the importance of adequate preparation of children for hospital admission and surgery.

The factors that adversely affect a child's emotional experience of hospital admission are shown in table 9.1.

Duration of hospital stay for children is shortened if their parents stay with them.[7] The factors in table 9.1 have all been shown to have a detrimental effect on the child's emotional experience of hospital admission. Children have different needs to adults.[8] The most important factor differentiating the needs of children from those of adults is their level of physical and psychological development.

CHILD'S-EYE VIEW OF THE OR

Children are smaller and less developed physically and emotionally than adults, so cannot see things adults see, or they see things differently. The operating room (OR) looks very different to a child than to an adult, and what adults can see and rationalise as necessary pieces of equipment can look very frightening to small children.

The paediatric OR must be planned around this concept. The OR reception area is a 'child-friendly' place, with pictures and cartoons on the walls, bright curtains and hangings, and colourful mobiles. Pictures on walls are at heights children can see: at the bottom of walls for children who walk into the

---

Table 9.1
Factors that adversely affect a child's emotional experience of hospital admission[6]

- Child's age
- Personality variations
- Painful and/or traumatic illnesses or injuries
- Inadequate preparation for routine admissions
- Previous admission experiences
- Parents not present
- Lack of paediatric training for staff
- Highly anxious parents
- Punishing parental style
- Length of stay

OR, and some higher up for children who come on a trolley. Toys, books, television and videotapes are provided as the children often do not have premedication and play on the floor until taken into the theatre. Parents should stay with their child until the child is anaesthetised, either in induction rooms or in the operating theatre itself. Some hospitals have toy cars for children to ride in from the ward to the OR, others have trolleys dressed up as boats or other 'fun' vehicles. Children often come into the OR in their own pyjamas or clothes.

MODELS OF CARE

With research about the emotional effect of hospital on children various modes involving parents and family in the hospitalised child's care have evolved and have been embraced, at least in theory, by children's hospitals in developed countries. However, in practice, they are not so widely accepted,[9] and further education is needed to convince health professionals of their worth. Total acceptance of parental involvement is often only an ideal not easily reached because it is difficult to remove judgmental attitudes from practice.[10] This is as relevant for the OR as for other departments and clinical areas within a hospital.

Various models of paediatric care exist, and all involve the parents. Arguably, the most common is family-centred care (FCC), though research suggests that while it has been accepted in theory, it is not fully practised.[9] While no one definition of FCC exists, it means that when a child is admitted to hospital, care should be planned around the whole family rather than the individual child, as all the family is inevitably affected by the admission of a child. Darbyshire[11] suggested that FCC is difficult to implement because parents feel that they are 'parenting in public' because the nurses are watching what they do, while nurses feel they are 'nursing in public' because of the parents' presence. He suggested that for FCC to succeed, understanding, empathetic communication between parents and nurses was necessary. This is particularly pertinent when a child is admitted to the OR because the parents and family are always anxious about their child having surgery.

Parents' wishes about their involvement in the care of their children in the OR are not always met.[12] Parental presence during anaesthetic induction is most often at the discretion of the anaesthetist, while presence in the PPACU (Paediatric Post-Anaesthetic Care Unit or Paediatric Recovery Room) is most often dependent on the nursing staff. Hospital policy may prevent parents being present in the operating theatres or PPACU. Reasons given for excluding parents from the PPACU often include the argument that too much can go wrong. Physical factors such as the bed area and availability of staff are used as reasons not to include parents. While these reasons may sound obstructionist, the reality is that a visit to a busy PPACU, where many unconscious children are admitted in quick succession following short operations such as myringotomy, would show that extra people in the room may indeed inhibit safe working practices. In such instances, privacy of individual children may be compromised, thereby lowering the quality of care being delivered. Hospital recovery rooms should be constructed to ensure that parents can accompany their children without compromising either the safety or privacy of child patients.

PRESENCE OF PARENTS

Until the 1960s, parents were often excluded from a hospital during a child's admission,[13] and while this has changed so that parents are now encouraged and often expected to stay for the duration of the child's admission, parental presence in the OR is a more contentious issue. Many hospitals and anaesthetists now encourage parental presence during anaesthetic induction (PPI), which is beneficial to the child,[14,15] and parents' and children's anxiety is ameliorated.[16–18] Empirical studies show this.[19–21] Parents must be well prepared by ensuring that they know what their child will look like as he/she becomes unconscious, that they are told everything that will happen, and that they must be escorted out of the theatre and assured that everything went well. There is little published about the presence of parents in the PPACU and more research is needed in this area.

PLAY

Play is an important therapeutic tool for hospitalised children and can be used to alleviate a child's fears about impending surgery. Routine play is necessary for children in hospital[22] as through play, a child maintains a normal perspective on living, thus reducing anxiety. He/she communicates ideas, copes with new perceptions, recognises feelings, decreases fear, clarifies distortions and comprehends threatening occurrences. Play helps children develop mastery over adverse situations. Through play, teachers, nurses and other health staff can handle a child's aggressive and hostile behaviour and help children prepare for impending situations such as operations. Hospitals should appoint a qualified adult to act as play leader,[23] and the play leader/therapist is an important part of the OR team.[24]

Clowns,[25] puppet shows[26] and theatre entertainers[27] are used to make hospitals more enjoyable places for children and they can be used in the OR. Music therapy offers opportunities for structured social interaction, for enhancement of education, for decreasing fear and anxiety, as distraction for painful procedures, as relaxation therapy, and for pain control.[28–30]

PREPARATION FOR THE OR

There is a large literature in both nursing and early childhood studies about the importance of preparation of young children for hospital, and nowhere is it more important than for the OR. Preadmission programmes were in place in hospitals in the USA in the 1970s.[31] To prepare children for surgery, explain the reason for the operation, interview the family, give written information, and facilitate discussions between nurses, doctors and parents. Information should be age appropriate and operations should never be suggested as a threat. Preparation processes and storybooks of children having surgery help prepare a child,[32] and all written material and discussions must be in the language of the patient. In the UK, Action for Sick Children published a book describing the importance of preparing children for hospital and medical procedures, and described ways to do so.[33] Community health workers, in liaison with schoolteachers, can prepare primary and preschool children for surgery by educating them about hospitalisation.[34] Calico dolls on which children can draw their impression of what is happening to them are therapeutic tools,[35] while some dolls are available that show the child the inner workings of

the body and make explanations easier and more valuable. Hospital play centres have areas set up with hospital beds and equipment so children can act out their own experiences.

In an evaluation of preparation of children's preday surgery admissions, the quality of the child's previous medical experiences influenced the child's anxiety levels for subsequent medical interventions. Children who had a previous negative experience were more anxious than children with positive or neutral experiences.[36]

SAFETY ISSUES FOR CHILDREN IN THE OR

Lee-Anne Waterman

Paediatric anaesthesia has developed because children are not 'little adults' and anaesthetics that are suitable for adults may not be so for children or infants. Their relative size and developmental stages are vitally important factors when undertaking the care of a child patient, be it for a major or minor procedure.

There are several safety considerations in relation to the size and developmental stage of children admitted to the OR.

CHECK-IN

Generally, it is considered (depending on local and hospital law) that under 18 years of age, a child requires a parent or legal guardian to be present for the purpose of informed consent and to ensure accurate identification of the child. The perioperative nurse recognises that patient advocacy is an important part of the role and has particular relevance for paediatrics. Particular attention must be paid to the following.

Right procedure

Consent – the operation to be performed must have been fully explained to the parent/guardian and child (where appropriate) and signed for by both that person and the surgeon (according to local policy). Laws about the legality of children signing their own consent form differ from country to country, but for the older child's feelings of autonomy, it is often a good idea to have him/her sign the form in conjunction with their parent/guardian. When the child is checked in, the parent is asked to state their understanding of the operation their child is having, and on what part of the body. The parent's explanation must agree with the documentation of the consent form. If there is some discrepancy, the doctors must ensure the parents are fully informed and the consent form signed again. If a parent has questions or needs more information, then this must be arranged as quickly as possible preoperatively. Any relevant X-rays should be taken into the OR with the child.

Right patient

Identification – according to local hospital policy, the child must have an identification band or label securely attached to his/her body. It must state accurately, as a minimum, the child's name, date of birth, any allergies and weight. This identification must agree fully with the child's other documentation such as hospital notes and consent form, and the parent must confirm the identity of the child with the nurse in the OR reception. In situations where a child is unaccompanied by a parent/guardian, then the person accompanying the child assumes this responsibility and must determine that legal consent has been obtained.

FASTING

The nurse must check with the parent the time the child last ate or drank, and what was ingested. While parents may have been informed of fasting times, sometimes the child will have been given a drink or snack because the parent may not fully understand the reasons for fasting.

If a child has consumed food or fluid, this information must be communicated as early as possible to the anaesthetist.

Loose teeth, the presence of any infections such as a runny nose or sores, recent contact with infectious diseases, rashes, allergies, any medications taken that day or any regular medication (particularly those due during the child's time in the OR), the presence of intravenous (IV) access devices, vital signs and, if necessary, an accurate fluid balance must be documented and brought to the attention of the anaesthetic, surgical and nursing staff who will continue the child's care intraoperatively.

SAFETY DURING ANAESTHETIC INDUCTION

Induction is commenced inside the perioperative suite with or without the parent present depending on local policy and the circumstances of the procedure. In cases where a 'rapid sequence anaesthetic' is required, it is often considered inappropriate to have parents present. As a result, this may be the first time the child has been alone in a frightening environment. It is important for a nurse to stay with the child at all times, talking to and comforting them. If a parent is accompanying a child through this phase, then their safety must also be considered. Many parents can feel anxious, distressed or even faint in the suite. Measures should be taken to reduce the amount of extraneous noise associated with setting up for procedures and preparing the theatre for the operation.

Specific safety issues for children at induction include the following.

- Keep bed rails and cot sides up at all times, and ensure a nurse or parent stays with the child to prevent falls from trolleys or theatre beds.
- Secure IV lines, arterial lines and epidural catheter lines safely and appropriately for the child's age and according to hospital policy.
- Check that any airway is appropriately secured.
- Connect the child to monitoring equipment, particularly oxygen saturation, electrocardiogram (ECG) and blood pressure, as quickly as possible once the child is asleep. A child with a dislodged tube or any other obstruction will desaturate and become bradycardic within seconds.
- Body temperature needs to be controlled with warm blankets, swaddling or the use of a warmer that can be used intraoperatively. Neonates and smaller children in particular lose body heat quickly and attention to keeping them warm at this stage is important.
- Children at risk of latex sensitivity or allergy need to be identified and latex-free equipment used according to local policy and practice.

INTRAOPERATIVE SAFETY ISSUES

Continuing from the induction phase, specific safety issues for children include the following.

- Pay on-going attention to body temperature by using body warmers and room temperature control. Warmed skin preparation, warmed wash solutions and warm IV solutions should be used when appropriate. Care must be taken not to overheat or burn the child while using these measures.
- Apply the diathermy plate carefully and correctly, ensuring the correct size for the weight of the child and positioning on a fleshy part of the body, e.g. thigh, abdomen or lower back. When applying the skin preparation, take care that fluid does not pool underneath or around the body. For volatile liquids and electrosurgical safety, see Chapter 6.
- Remove all metal nappy pins, metal buttons and press-studs to prevent possible burns caused by subsequent diathermy (for electrosurgery, see Chapter 6).
- Carefully and accurately measure blood and fluid losses, report them to the anaesthetist and document them on a fluid record sheet. Used swabs (preweighed while dry) should be weighed to ascertain blood loss, particularly with infants, and paediatric sucker catchment bottles with millilitre measurements should be used. The blood volume of a healthy 10 kg infant is approximately 800 ml (10 ml kg^{-1}),[37] and a blood loss of 200 ml would equal one-quarter of the child's total volume.
- Pay close attention to the positioning of equipment and scrub staff at the operating table once the patient has been draped.
- Ensure that protective equipment such as a lead apron is placed over the child who requires X-ray intraoperatively, e.g. children having central lines inserted or fractures manipulated.
- Position the child on the operating table as discussed in Chapter 4. Particular paediatric positions require special safety considerations, e.g. the 'flying foetus' position used in craniofacial surgery, which involves lying the child prone, neck extended and face facing out. Too much extension can lead to venous congestion from blood pooling at the back of the neck. Once the child is anaesthetised, it is placed prone on a special beanbag, which is moulded to shape and the air extracted. At this point, there must be no ridges or wrinkles that will cause pressure.

- Drains and indwelling catheters must be secured carefully. Young children, when awake or when regaining consciousness, will often try to remove or pull out tubes that frighten or cause them discomfort.

POSTANAESTHETIC/POSTOPERATIVE

Postanaesthesia is a continuation of the perioperative phase. Each hospital has its own process for moving patients out of the OR and into the Paediatric Post-Anaesthesia Care Unit (PPACU). According to each hospital's guidelines, children are moved from the OR to the PPACU in various anaesthetic stages ranging from fully ventilated to extubated and rousable. Special considerations for children in this phase include the following.

- Place the child on a paediatric recovery trolley and ensure the side rails are up. In particular, ensure the head is not hyperextended. Children have short, narrow airways that are easily obstructed as a result of extension or occlusion, e.g. swelling, mucus and vomit, and are particularly susceptible to irritation, e.g. laryngospasm.
- Oxygen, mask and T-piece, and suction must be immediately available and saturation monitoring attached once the child arrives in the PPACU. An obstructed airway or apnoea in a child can result in sudden respiratory arrest.
- It is important that a child is never left alone on a bed or trolley in the PPACU. Many times, small children will wake up in the unfamiliar area, possibly experiencing pain and often being hungry, thirsty, confused and frightened. They will jump, fall or crawl off beds that do not have adequate safety rails and an adult (nurse or parent) should be with them at all times.
- IV access and IV lines must be secured as quickly as possible using arm boards and taping. Small children in particular often will not tolerate IV lines and attempt to pull them out. The same is true for drains such as indwelling catheters and wound drains. Secure taping with splints will ensure the IV lines cannot be dislodged, and constant watching by an adult is needed to ensure the newly wakened child does not pull drains and other tubing out.

- Distressed, confused children who are not fully awake can hurt themselves by self-harming behaviour such as scratching their faces or other body parts.
- Arm splints may be ordered and required for some children such as babies who have had palate or lip surgery. These also need to be applied as quickly as possible, ideally before the child has woken up.
- A child whose limb is splinted for safe IV access or to prevent them harming operation sites must have the circulation in their limb checked regularly.
- Ongoing monitoring of body temperature is important. Hypothermia will cause periodic breathing, apnoea and delays in rousing a postoperative child.
- Ongoing and accurate monitoring of fluid intake and losses from drips, drains and dressing.

STANDING ORDERS

Because of the independent nature of nursing work in the PPACU, standing orders are often designed to provide guidelines from which nurses can work. To be legally binding, these must be written in conjunction with the anaesthetist in charge of the PPACU and are most often designed by a committee comprised of the head anaesthetist, nurse in charge of the PPACU and, if different, the nurse in charge of the OR. A sample of standing orders for the postoperative recovery of children who have had adenotonsillectomy is shown in table 9.2.

Table 9.2
Standing orders for a child postadenotonsillectomy

In the postoperative phase, a child with obstructive sleep apnoea (OSA) that has also had an ear, nose and throat (ENT) procedure is at risk due to postoperative swelling and oedema. The patient should be closely monitored for signs of respiratory failure in addition to routine postoperative observation.

Postoperative oxygen standing orders

If a child's oxygen saturations drop to <90%:

(1) Rouse the child.
(2) Give oxygen if required.
(3) If the child is unrousable, commence resuscitation as per the code procedure.
(4) Call the consultant or registrar concerned.
(5) 'Special' the child until reviewed by medical staff.

Note that the child must not be left unattended with oxygen *in situ* while awaiting medical review.

Postoperative pain relief orders for 'not for narcotic' children

It may be necessary for a child to be ordered narcotic pain relief and very close observation must then be undertaken for a minimum of 2 hours postadministration. The child should be on pulse oximetry, and visual observation should include rousability and respiratory rate.

 If a 'Not-for-Narcotic' child is in pain and requires stronger pain relief than ordered:

(1) Call the ENT consultant or registrar concerned for a review of respiratory status and pain relief order.
(2) Give pain relief as ordered.
(3) Monitor oxygen saturations, respiratory rate and depth and rousability:
  - 5 minutely for 15 min
  - 15 minutely for 2 h.
(4) If oxygen saturation drops to <90%:
  - Rouse the child.
  - Give oxygen as required.
  - If unrousable, commence resuscitation as per the code procedure.
  - Call the ENT registrar or consultant concerned.
  - 'Special' the child until medical review.

References

1. Jessner L, Blom GE, Waldfogel S. Emotional implications of tonsillectomy and adenoidectomy on children. *Psychoanal Study Child* 1952; 7: 126–169.

2. Blom GE. The reactions of hospitalized children to illness. *Pediatrics* 1958; 22: 590–600.

3. Oremland EK, Oremland JD. *The Effects of Hospitalization on Children: Models for their Care.* Springfield: Charles C. Thomas, 1973.

4. Lansdown R. The psychological health status of children in hospital. *J Roy Soc Med* 1992; 85: 125–126.

5. Strachan RG. Emotional responses to paediatric hospitalization. *Nurs Times* 1993; 89: 45–49.

6. Wright MC. Behavioural effects of hospitalization in children. *J Paediatr Child Health* 1995; 31: 165–167.

7. Taylor MRH, O'Connor P. Resident parents and shorter hospital stay. *Arch Dis Child* 1989; 64: 274–276.

8. Price S. The special needs of children. *J Adv Nurs* 1994; 20: 227–232.

9. Shields L. A comparative study of the care of hospitalized children in developed and developing countries. PhD thesis, University of Queensland, 1999.

10. Darbyshire P. *Living with a Sick Child in Hospital: The Experiences of Parents and Nurses.* London: Chapman & Hall, 1994.

11. Darbyshire P. Family-centred care within contemporary British paediatric nursing. *Br J Nurs* 1995; 4: 31–33.

12. Alsop-Shields L. Perioperative care of children in a transcultural context. *AORN J* 2000; 71: 1004–1020.

13. Shields L, Nixon J. I want my mummy – changes in the care of children in hospital. *Collegian* 1998; 5: 16–19.

14. *A Recommended Policy Relating to the Provision of Care for Children Undergoing Anaesthesia.* Sydney: Association for the Welfare of Children in Hospital, 1989.

15. Burns LS. Advances in pediatric anesthesia. *Nurs Clin North Am* 1997; 32: 45–71.

16. Schulman JL, Foley JM, Vernon MA, Allan D. A study of the effect of the mother's presence during anaesthesia induction. *Pediatrics* 1967; 39: 111–114.

17. LaRosa-Nash PA, Murphy JM. A clinical case study: parent–present induction of anesthesia in children. *Pediatr Nurs* 1996; 22: 109–111.

18. Landers H. Anaesthesia induction: should parents be present? *Info Nursing* 1994; 25: 10–12.

19. Smerling AJ, Lieberman I, Rothstein P. Parents' presence during the induction of anesthesia in children: parents' viewpoint. *Anesthesiology* 1988; 69: A743.

20. LaRosa-Nash PA, Murphy JM. An approach to pediatric perioperative care: parent-present induction. *Nurs Clin North Am* 1997; 32: 183–199.

21. Cameron JA, Bond MJ, Pointer SC. Reducing the anxiety of children undergoing surgery: parental presence during anaesthetic induction. *J Paediatr Child Health* 1996; 32: 51–56.

22. Petrillo M, Sanger S. *Emotional Care of Hospitalized Children: An Environmental Approach.* Philadelphia: Lippincott, 1972.

23. Hart D. The role of the play leader in hospital. *Aust Nurs J* 1976; 5: 30–32.

24. *Hospital: A Deprived Environment for Children – The Case for Hospital Play Schemes.* London: Save the Children, 1989.

25. Simonds C. Clowning in hospitals is no joke. *Children in Hospital* 1995; 21: 3–4.

26. Haris S. College students bring puppet shows to children in hospital. *Children in Hospital* 1995; 21: 5–6.

27. Martin G. Once upon a time: the story of the Allsports Hospital Entertainers. *Children in Hospital* 1995; 21: 1–2.

28. Davis WB, Gfeller KE, Thaut MH. *An Introduction to Music Therapy: Theory and Practice.* Dubuque: Wm C. Brown, 1992.

29. Marley LS. The use of music with hospitalized infants and toddlers: a descriptive study. *J Mus Ther* 1984; 21: 125–132.

30. Aldridge K. The use of music to relieve pre-operational anxiety in children attending day surgery. *Aust J Mus Ther* 1993; 4: 19–35.

31. Johnson BH. Before hospitalization: a preparation program for the child and his family. *Child Today* 1974; November–December: 18–21.

32. Eckhardt LO, Prugh DG. Preparing children psychologically for painful medical and surgical procedures. In: Gellert E (ed) *Psychosocial Aspects of Pediatric Care.* New York: Grune & Stratton, 1978.

33. Rodin J. *Will this hurt? Preparing Children for Hospital and Medical Procedures.* London: NAWCH, 1989.

34. Johnson A. Children and their families in hospital. In: Clements A (ed.) *Infant and Family Health in Australia,* 2nd edn. Melbourne: Churchill Livingstone, 1992.

35. English C, Bond S. Evidence based nursing: easier said than done. *Paediatr Nurs* 1998; 10: 7–8, 10–11.

36. Dahlquist LM, Gil KM, Armstrong, D, DeLawyer DD, Greene P, Wuori D. Preparing children for medical examinations: the importance of previous medical experience. *Health Psychol* 1986; 5: 249–259.

37. Morgan GE, Mikhail MS. *Clinical Anesthesiology,* 2nd edn. Stamford: Appleton & Lange, 1996.

Psychosocial care of children in the perioperative area

10 | Surgical procedures on children

Annabel Herron, Linda Shields, Ann Tanner and Lee-Anne Waterman

Surgical procedures performed on the neonate, infant, child and adolescent are generally significantly different from those procedures performed on the adult. A child can be defined thus.

- Premature infant: born after a gestation period of less than 37 weeks.
- Neonate: born from 38 weeks' gestation to 28 days (1 month) old.
- Baby: from 1 month old to 12 months of age.
- Infant: a child in the first period of life.
- Child: a young person between infancy and adolescence.
- Adolescent: period of life from puberty to maturity terminating legally at the age of majority.

PSYCHOLOGICAL TRAUMA

Minimising psychological trauma to the child undergoing a surgical procedure is paramount for the paediatric perioperative nurse. Children are very vulnerable in the hospital environment and this should be foremost in the minds of the nursing staff in the OR. Important factors that influence the care of the child in the OR include the child's age and temperament, the operative site, the nature and extent of the surgery being performed, the degree and duration of postoperative discomfort, and the length of stay in hospital. These vary between children and the amount of confidence the child has in those who care for them is of utmost importance. Great effort should be made to minimise psychological disturbances in children undergoing surgery.

There are many and varied ways of reducing psychological trauma to the child. Use methods of distraction to take the focus away from the fact that the child is in an unfamiliar and frightening environment. Play games with children, point out pictures in the room and ask questions of the children so they do not notice what is going on around them. These methods are age-related; the older child will require explanations and more detail of procedures being performed. Always be honest when children require answers, as there is no point telling them that something will not hurt if it will. Loss of trust between the nurse and their patient makes a job very difficult. How the child's questions are handled is just as important as the factual content of the answers. Deal with possible sources of fear, and emphasise the pleasant aspects of an operative experience, e.g. how good they will feel for having faced the situation bravely, and how they will have many stories to tell their friends. Adjust the amount and type of information to the child's age and particular needs; older children will expect more details. These methods are useful tools to use in the paediatric operating theatre and with time become second nature to the paediatric perioperative nurse.

ROLE OF THE PARENT

The child's parents require much consideration while their child in hospital, and particularly when their child requires surgery. Some children need surgery on their first day of life, and these parents require a lot of care and concern. Other parents have not been separated from their children at all and will be upset and frightened for the safety of their children. Support and reassurance must be given to the family of the child undergoing an operative procedure. They need a full and comprehensive understanding of procedures to be performed on their child as informed consent is given by the parents and a signed consent form is a legal requirement before the child enters the operating room (OR). Some paediatric operating theatre suites have induction or anaesthetic rooms available that enable parents to be present during the beginning of the anaesthetic. This is often a good way of alleviating anxiety, not only for the child, but also for the parents.

COMMON SURGICAL PROCEDURES PERFORMED ON CHILDREN

The same types of instruments are used for surgery on children as on adults. However, paediatric instruments are often smaller and more delicate with less pronounced curves and are lighter in weight. The smaller the child, the smaller the instrument the surgeon is likely to use. Laparoscopic surgery is becoming popular in the paediatric setting,[1] and the size of instruments is an important consideration for ease of use and evaluation shows it to be a cost-efficient alternative to regular procedures.[2]

Paediatric surgery, like adult surgery, is divided into areas of speciality. These specialities include the following: general, ear, nose and throat (ENT), neurosurgery, urology, orthopaedics, ophthalmology, and plastic and craniofacial surgery. Paediatric general surgery includes chest and abdominal problems in neonates, infants, children and adolescents. Some common surgical procedures performed on children are explained in further detail.

ABDOMINAL PAEDIATRIC SURGERY

Appendicectomy

Appendicitis is a common, important and sometimes fatal disease in childhood.[3] Consequently, an appendicectomy (or appendectomy in North American parlance) is a relatively common paediatric procedure. The appendix can be removed either by an incisional, open operation or, more recently, by laparoscopy. In both procedures, the appendix is located, tied off from its stump and excised, and each surgeon has a specific method of doing this. The abdominal cavity is then washed out and closed.

Perioperative nursing implications

- The child will receive a general anaesthetic.
- The child will lie supine on the operating table.
- The child will require a patient return electrode/diathermy plate.
- A basic laparotomy set of instruments will be used.
- Peritoneal cavity may require washing out with normal saline before the abdomen is closed.

Atresia

'Atresia' means 'the absence of a normal body opening, duct or canal ...'[4] (p. 144). Intestinal atresias occur most frequently in the ileum, but can also occur in the duodenum, jejunum or colon. Intestinal atresia can be found by ultrasound during pregnancy, or on the first or second day of life, when the abdomen becomes distended, the infant fails to pass stools and, finally, begins to vomit, all signs of gut obstruction. Radiological examination will detect the deformity. Other common atresias are oesophageal (OA) and tracheal. A tracheal atresia will often involve the oesophagus, forming a tracheo-oesphageal fistula (TOF), where there is a common passage joining the trachea and oesophagus.[5] OA and TOF are related conditions found in the neonate, usually detected soon after birth by the inability to pass a nasogastric catheter into the oesophagus.[6] These conditions are of unknown aetiology, but occur in early fetal life.

As OA is lethal, operative repair is done as soon as possible after detection. A thoracotomy incision is performed and the defects repaired with anastomosis of the oesophageal ends. If a TOF exists, repair will include ligature of the tracheal branch.[6] Repair of OA or TOF may require repeated operations over many years.[7]

Perioperative nursing implications

- The child will receive a general anaesthetic.
- The child will lie supine on the operating table.
- The child will require a patient return electrode/diathermy plate.
- A basic laparotomy set of instruments will be used requiring extra retractors for the chest, ligating clips, dilators, vessel loops and an infant chest drain.

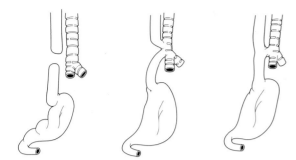

Fig. 10.1 Atresias: structures of tracheo-oesophageal fistulae

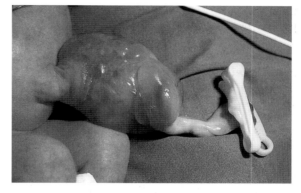

Fig. 10.2 Omphalocele with the abdominal organs protruding through the child's umbilicus

- Warming mattress will be required, the temperature of the room set high and fluids warmed.

Gastroschisis and omphalocele

Gastroschisis and omphalocele are similar conditions found at birth, the aetiology of which is poorly understood. Gastroschisis is the herniation of abdominal contents through the abdominal wall lateral to a normal umbilical cord, while an omphalocele is a congenital malformation in which the intestines protrude from the abdominal wall and are covered by a sac from which the umbilical cord begins.

These defects are often detected by ultrasound before birth, and it is unusual for a child born with gastroschisis to have other serious birth defects. However, undescended testis is common in these children. Omphalocele, on the other hand, is often associated with chromosome abnormalities, which include syndromes such as Beckwith–Wiedemann and Down's syndromes.[8] Rupture of the omphalocele constitutes an emergency requiring immediate surgery.

Operative treatment depends on the severity of the condition, its size and the health of the infant. A simple closure is rarely possible as the organs have to be pushed back into the abdomen. Often a series of operations over many years is necessary. To prevent increased pressure in the abdomen, a pouch or 'silo' of Silastic™ sheeting is often used to contain the gut and over a period, as gravity allows the organs to fall

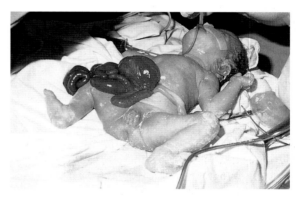

Fig. 10.3 Gastroschisis, with the abdominal organs protruding lateral to the umbilicus. Note the visible stomach, bowel and fallopian tubes

back into the infant's growing abdominal cavity, the pouch is shortened until it can be removed and the abdominal wall closed.[9] In the case of omphaloceles with large openings, surgery may be contraindicated, and these lesions are allowed to epithelialise over a long period.[10]

Perioperative nursing implications

- The child will receive a general anaesthetic.
- The child will lie supine on the operating table.
- The child will require a patient return electrode/diathermy plate.
- A basic laparotomy set of instruments will be used.
- Sterile Silastic™ sheets must be available.

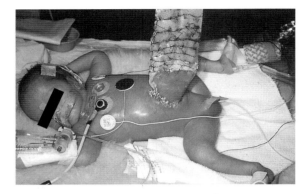

Fig. 10.4 Surgical reduction of an omphalocele. The 'silo' contains the infant's abdominal contents for the treatment of omphalocele

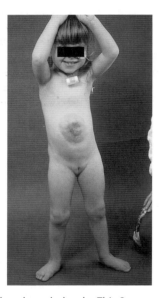

Fig. 10.5 Closed omphalocele. This 3-year-old girl was born with a large omphalocele, which was allowed to epithelialise. Eventually epithelial tissue grew to cover the abdominal organs.

Imperforate anus

Imperforate anus is the absence of a normal anal opening. Clinically, it is divided into three main categories: 1. low anomalies, occur when most of the rectum has developed normally and sphincters are present, but the anus itself is non-existent, 2. Intermediate anomalies consist of those where the rectum ends at or below the level of the *puborectalis* muscle without passing into an anal passage and high anomalies occur when the rectum ends above the *puborectalis* muscle, and the internal and external sphincters are absent. Genitourinary fistulae usually occur with high anomalies.[7] Diagnosis is usually made shortly after birth when routine physical examination reveals no anal opening, or when a neonate fails to pass meconium stool in the first 24–48 hours after birth. Imperforate anus occurs in about 1 in 5000 births and its cause is unknown.[11]

Surgical treatment of infants with imperforate anus depends upon the severity of the condition and can range from a simple perineal anoplasty to make a passage in the perineum for the anus, to complicated procedures for the reconstruction of bowel, vagina and urethral walls. Colostomy is often part of the operative procedures for high anomalies.

Perioperative nursing implications

- The child will receive a general anaesthetic.
- The child will be lying supine on the operating table with legs taped into a lithotomy position in order to operate on the perineum.
- The child will require a patient return electrode/diathermy plate.
- A basic laparotomy set of instruments will be used with the addition of anal retractors, dilators and lubricant gel, and a nerve and muscle stimulator.

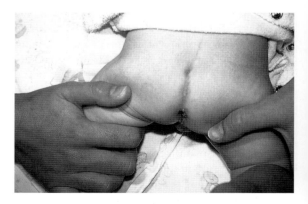

Fig. 10.6 Imperforate anus

- The child may require an indwelling catheter to be inserted during the procedure.

Hernia

A hernia is the protrusion of an organ through an abnormal opening in the muscle wall of a body cavity.[4] Two types of hernia found in children are umbilical and inguinal. Umbilical hernias are of small clinical consequence and usually resolve spontaneously; usually they are repaired for cosmetic reasons.[12] Operative repair is often done in day surgery or as an outpatient procedure, often with a caudal anaesthetic block.[13] Inguinal hernia is common in children, but has more serious consequences than umbilical hernia. A loop of intestine enters the inguinal canal and can become obstructed, and strangulation of the hernia can occur.[4]

Inguinal hernias account for about 80% of all hernias and are the most common surgical procedures done in infancy. These hernias appear more frequently in boys than in girls. Repair consists of repairing the protrusion in the hernial sac and anchoring it in the inguinal canal.[5] Inguinal hernia can be associated with hydrocele.

Perioperative nursing implications

- The child will receive a general anaesthetic.
- The child will be lying supine on the operating table.

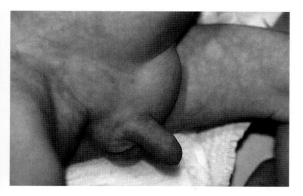

Fig. 10.7 Hernia. This child has bilateral inguinal hernias

- The child will require a patient return electrode / diathermy plate.
- A basic minor set of instruments will be used.

Intussusception

Intussusception is the telescoping of one segment of bowel into the lumen of another[4] and is one of the most common causes of gut obstruction in infancy.[7] About 80% of intussusceptions are in the ileocolic region of the bowel.[14] It can occur at any age but is most frequently seen in children between 5 and 10 months of age, and 70% of them are male. As the bowel telescopes, it becomes compressed, resulting in oedema of the bowel wall, compromised circulation and, if left untreated, strangulation of the gut.

Treatment begins with insertion of a nasogastric tube to deflate the stomach, and insertion of an IV line and fluid administration. It is sometimes possible to correct the invagination of the loops of bowel using barium or air under radiological control. If this is unsuccessful, or the intussusception recurs, surgery will be required to access the affected bowel

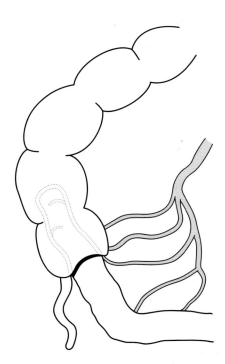

Fig. 10.8 Intussusception

and massage it back into normal alignment; or, if the bowel has been damaged, removal of affected areas may be necessary.[14] An appendicectomy is usually done at the same time because the site of the scar is often the same as that for an appendicectomy. In later life, if the person presents with abdominal pain and an 'appendix' scar, treatment for appendicitis may be delayed.[14]

Perioperative nursing implications

- The child will receive a general anaesthetic.
- The child will be placed supine on the operating table.
- The child will require a patient return electrode/diathermy plate.
- A basic minor set of instruments will be used with the addition of some retractors.

Necrotizing enterocolitis (NEC)

The evidence of NEC has increased with technological advances which support the lives of infants born prematurely, as over 90% of children with NEC are premature newborns.[15] The cause of NEC is unknown, and suggestions include immaturity of bowel wall function and motility,[16] hypoxia and infection, and there has been a suggested link between NEC and infant formula feeding,[7] while breast milk is thought to provide some protection against it.[17,18] However, all these are speculative and more research is needed to clarify all the issues.[19]

The infant presents with abdominal distension and bloody stools soon after enteral feeding has begun. Diagnosis is based on the clinical picture and radiological review. Treatment can be either medical, which involves nasogastric suction, and antibiotics; or surgical (required in up to 50% of cases) to repair perforation or severe necrosis of the gut.[16]

Perioperative nursing implications

- The child will receive a general anaesthetic.
- The child will be lying supine on the operating table.
- The child will require a patient return electrode/diathermy plate.
- A major laparotomy set of instruments will be used with the addition of bowel clamps such as Debakey clamps.

Pyloric stenosis

Pyloric stenosis is a commonly seen paediatric condition and is caused by thickening of the gastric outlet musculature, although the aetiology of this is unknown.[7] It occurs in up to three infants per 1000, and is more common in males than in females.[20] Its characteristic presentation of projectile vomiting in a previously well infant and visible peristalsis on the abdominal wall makes clinical diagnosis simple, though varying degrees of these symptoms can cloud the issue and X-ray or ultrasound can be used to confirm the findings.[20] Surgery to open the thickened pylorus (pyloromyotomy or Ramstedt's operation) involves splitting the muscle fibres[9] to ensure free passage of food into the duodenum.

Perioperative nursing implications

- The child will receive a general anaesthetic.
- The child will be lying supine on the operating table.
- The child will require a patient return electrode/diathermy plate.
- A basic minor set of instruments will be used with the addition of a hernia director that some surgeons prefer to split the pylorus.

GENITOURINARY PAEDIATRIC SURGERY

Circumcision

Circumcision is one of the oldest operations and provokes much controversy.[21,22] Sometimes it is done because a specific problem with the foreskin

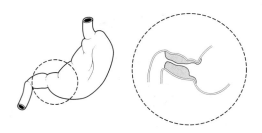

Fig. 10.9 Pyloric stenosis: thickened muscle in the pylorus

(prepuce) exists; other times it is done for family, cultural or religious reasons. Although routine circumcision was once advocated for all newborn males, current feeling is that it is not necessary, as an understanding and performance of hygiene has improved in modem times. As with all surgery, it carries some risks to the child and complications, such as penile adhesions,[23] and inconspicuous penis[24] occur.

Clinical indicators for circumcision include narrowing at the tip of the penis (phimosis), infections (posthitis, balanitis)[13,25] or paraphimosis, where the prepuce cannot be returned to its normal position after being retracted down the glans.[13]

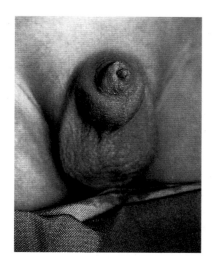

Fig. 10.12 Circumcision: 'inconspicuous' penis

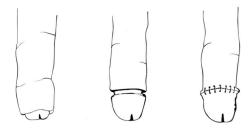

Fig. 10.10 Circumcision: procedure for circumcision

The procedure, if done on older boys, involves a general anaesthetic and the foreskin is lifted, excised and rejoined to the shaft skin. Neonatal circumcision, on which debate rages, is usually done with local anaesthetic, often with devices that include a bell-shaped arrangement around which the foreskin is cut away. Complications of neonatal circumcision include bleeding and infection, though the incidence of these is low.[25]

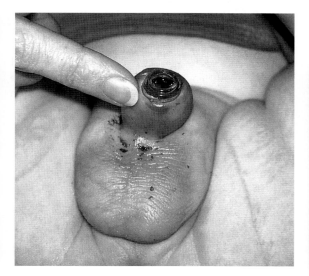

Fig. 10.11 Circumcision: bleeding following circumcision

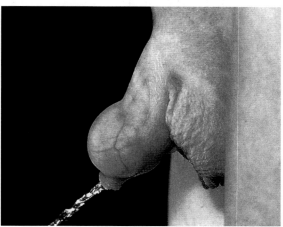

Fig. 10.13 Phimosis

Perioperative nursing implications

- The child will receive a general anaesthetic and sometimes a caudal block.
- The child will be lying supine on the operating table.
- The child will require a patient return electrode/diathermy plate.
- A basic minor set of instruments will be used.

Hydrocele

A hydrocele is a collection of fluid around the testicle, which occurs in infants when the canal between the peritoneal cavity and the scrotum fails to close during fetal development.[4] The condition often resolves spontaneously, but sometimes requires surgical intervention. Hydroceles are often related to inguinal hernias and the surgical procedure for their repair is similar, with drainage of the fluid in the sac.[9]

Perioperative nursing implications

- The child will receive a general anaesthetic and sometimes a caudal block.
- The child will be lying supine on the operating table.

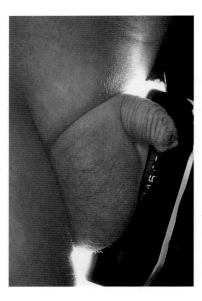

Fig. 10.14 Hydrocele

- The child will require a patient return electrode/diathermy plate.
- A basic minor set of instruments will be used.

Undescended testicles (orchidopexy)

If the testis does not descend into the scrotum during fetal development, the infant may be born with an undescended testis. Some descend spontaneously in the first year of life, but to ensure that complications such as torsion of the testis and malignancy[26] do not occur later in life, the operation known as 'orchidopexy' is performed. The procedure involves finding the testis in the groin (made easier by a laparoscope), pulling it down into the scrotal sac and anchoring it there.[13]

Perioperative nursing implications

- The child will receive a general anaesthetic and sometimes a caudal block.
- The child will be lying supine on the operating table.
- The child will require a patient return electrode/diathermy plate.
- A basic minor set of instruments will be used.

Hypospadias repair

Some boys are born with their urinary meatus situated somewhere along the shaft of their penis, rather than at its tip. The incidence is about 1 in every 125 live male births[27] and the incidence is said to be increasing in many countries,[28] with many suggestions about why this is so including exposure to environmental factors,[29,30] though this is debated by others.[31,32]

Repair depends on the position of the lesion and its size. Repair may take one operation, or many, and is usually done in the first year of life. The techniques used are many and varied, including the use of laser and tissue solder,[33] but their aim is always to place the urethral meatus in the tip of the penis, to correct curvature, to create a conical glans and to ensure cosmetic acceptability.[34]

Perioperative nursing implications

- The child will receive a general anaesthetic and sometimes a caudal block.

- The child will be lying supine on the operating table.
- The child will require a patient return electrode/diathermy plate.
- A basic minor set of instruments will be used.
- Dressings as per the surgeon's preference must be available as some can be very elaborate and time consuming.
- Have a urinary catheter available in the room.

SOME GENERAL PAEDIATRIC SURGICAL PROCEDURES

Diaphragmatic hernia

Diaphragmatic hernia occurs due to failed closure of the diaphragm in embryonic development.[35] The gut and other organs find their way through the defect and sit in the chest, displacing the heart and lungs. Prenatal diagnosis allows preparation for treatment after birth. This usually includes ventilation, as respiration can be seriously compromised, and ventilation must be maintained until the abnormality is surgically corrected and the child's chest grows to allow room for the correct placement of the organs. Once the baby's condition is stable, surgery can go ahead. Surgery may need to be done in stages depending on the severity and extent of the abnormality and its effect on the heart and lungs. However, its aim is to anchor the abdominal organs in the abdominal cavity and provide room for normal growth and function of the thoracic organs.

Perioperative nursing implications

- The child will receive a general anaesthetic.
- The child will be laid supine on the operating table.
- The child will require a patient return electrode/diathermy plate.
- A basic major laparotomy set of instruments will be used.
- Use of patient-warming equipment to prevent hypothermia is of utmost importance because of the length of surgical time.
- A chest drain and water seal drain will be required.
- Silastic™ sheeting or mesh may be required.

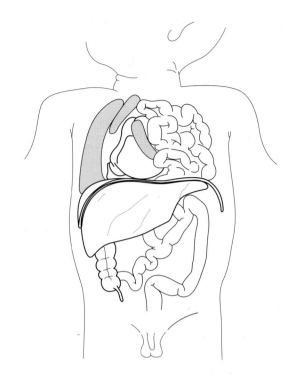

Fig. 10.15 Diaphragmatic hernia

Insertion of central venous line

A 'central line' is an intravenous catheter placed into a large, central vein such as the superior vena cava. A central line is needed to give the medical team access to a large vein that can be used to give fluids, including total parenteral nutrition, measure the amount of fluid in the body or give medication that might irritate smaller veins. Older children are sedated for the central line insertion; younger children are usually given a general anaesthetic. Central lines are usually inserted in the OR, though in some situations, insertion can be done at the bedside or in the treatment room.

Perioperative nursing implications

- The child will receive a general anaesthetic or, if old enough and cooperative, a local anaesthetic can be used.
- The child will be lying supine on the operating table with a sandbag under the shoulder if the line is to be placed in the clavicular area.

- The child will require a patient return electrode/diathermy plate.
- A basic minor set of instruments will be used with a tunnelling device.
- Have ampoules of heparin available.

Minimally invasive surgery

Minimally invasive surgery (MIS) using scopes, lights, monitors and cameras with specially designed instruments through several small incisions[36] can be used for a wide variety of operations in children, in whom it is particularly useful because of their small size and distress from pain and hospital admission.[37] It is used in a wide variety of paediatric surgical specialities such as cardiac surgery,[38] abdominal procedures,[39] oncology[40] and urology,[41] and is becoming widely accepted. In a survey of members of the American Pediatric Surgical Association published in 1998, 82% of paediatric surgeons who were surveyed were using minimally invasive procedures routinely.[42] It is safe, efficient and well tolerated by children and produces better cosmetic results than usual surgery, and has reduced length of stay in hospital[43] and a speedier return to school.[44]

Perioperative nursing implications

- The child will receive a general anaesthetic.
- The child will be lying supine on the operating table or in a lithotomy position for fundoplication surgery.
- The child will require a patient return electrode/diathermy plate.
- Laparoscopic instrumentation is required and the camera, monitor, CO_2 insufflator and light source must be in the OR.

Fetal surgery

MIS has allowed a new branch of paediatric surgery to develop – fetal surgery, where the uterus of the pregnant woman is opened and a defect in the fetus repaired.[45] Much of this work is still experimental using animal models[46] but has been used successfully for repair of defects such as myelomeningocele and hydrocephalus,[47,48] cardiac anomalies,[49] urological defects,[50] thoracic abnormalities that can

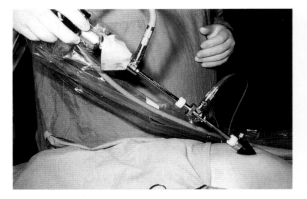

Fig. 10.16 Minimally invasive surgery: laparoscopic testicular localisation

obstruct respiration,[51] diaphragmatic hernia,[52] gut abnormalities,[53] and cleft lip and palate.[54] Scarring is greatly reduced in fetal surgery,[55] but the risk of premature birth is greatly increased,[45] so decisions have to be made after a careful risk–benefit analysis. Concern has begun to be voiced over the effects on the fetus, e.g. does it feel pain during surgery?[56] Topics for ethical debate on fetal surgery include the dilemma faced by women and their families who are offered this still risky option to repair what may be a lethal abnormality in their child, and choosing between fetal surgery and termination after an unfavourable prenatal diagnosis.

Perioperative nursing implications

- Two patients require surgery in this situation: the mother and the unborn child. Therefore, both must be considered when planning surgery.
- The mother will require a general anaesthetic.
- The mother will be lying supine on the operating table.
- The mother will require a patient return electrode/diathermy plate.
- Laparoscopic instrumentation and equipment are required involving a monitor and camera, a CO_2 insufflator and a light source.

EAR, NOSE AND THROAT (ENT) SURGERY

ENT surgery constitutes a major part of paediatric surgery as it treats some of the most common surgical illnesses such as otitis media, sinusitis, tonsillitis and adenoiditis, and upper airway obstruction. Most children for ENT surgery are admitted as day-stay patients as the operations are small, simple and quickly performed. They include adenoid and tonsillectomy, myringotomy, and insertion of grommets. A few are outlined here.

Tonsillectomy and adenoidectomy

There is some controversy over the need for tonsillectomy and adenoidectomy[7] with some suggestion that the operations are performed unnecessarily in some instances.[57] In children, adenotonsillectomy or adenoidectomy are performed to treat recurrent tonsillitis, obstruction of the nasopharynx and obstructive sleep apnoea.[58] Adenoidectomy can be performed by itself and is usually done to relieve pressure from inflamed adenoids on the middle ear.[59,60] Research has indicated that it is safe to perform adenoidectomy as out-patient or day-case surgery,[61] but risk of complications, in particular postoperative haemorrhage, prevent children having tonsillectomy from going home on the same day,[62–64] though this is contested.[65]

Traditionally, there have been two methods for tonsillectomy: using a tonsil snare (guillotine), which loops over the tonsil and cuts it off at its base,[66] and, more recently, by sharp or blunt dissection.[5] However, innovative methods are tried often with the main aims of decreasing bleeding and postoperative pain. New methods include tonsillotomy using a CO_2 laser,[67] using an ultrasonic scalpel[68] and cryoanalgesia.[69]

Perioperative nursing implications

- The child will receive a general anaesthetic.
- The child will be lying supine on the operating table.
- The child will require a patient return electrode/diathermy plate.
- A tonsillectomy set of instruments will be used that will include tonsil snares, adenatomes, and a mouth gag and blade.

Myringotomy and insertion of tympanostomy tubes (grommets)

Otitis media, where fluid builds up behind the eardrum, is very common and can take two forms in

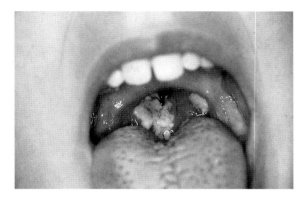

Fig. 10.17 Tonsillitis: the infected tonsils are covered with pus

children: acute and chronic. A short and open Eustachian tube predisposes young children to otitis media. Acute otitis media is a painful condition treated variously with nasal decongestant drops and antibiotics. Repeated, chronic episodes of otitis media often require surgical intervention.

Chronic suppurative otitis media and its variant, chronic serous otitis media, is a disease found most commonly in indigenous races of the world: Australian Aborigines,[70–72] Maori children,[73] Canadian Inuit[74] and American Indians,[75] to name but a few. It is a disease of particular importance for these children as their hearing is impaired and this negatively affects their school performance. It is treated by myringotomy, which affords proper hearing conduction by releasing fluid from behind the drum, and provides less scarring than if the drum were allowed to rupture spontaneously.

Myringotomy is a very common paediatric procedure in which a small incision is made into the tympanic membrane to release fluid and relieve pressure due to otitis media.[76] Sometimes myringotomy is done singly. At other times it is supplemented by the insertion of tubes (grommets), which equalise pressure on both sides of the ear drum, allowing free passage of sound waves to the inner ear. The grommets fall out as the ear grows, and in about 1% of patients a small hole is left that may later require repair by tympanoplasty.[77] Insertion of grommets takes about 10 minutes, so an operation list with a preponderance of these operations is usually very busy.

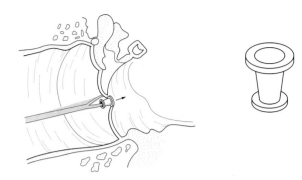

Fig. 10.18 Grommet insertion: the grommet (right) with insertion of the grommet into the myringotomy incision (left) (see arrow)

Perioperative nursing implications

- The child will receive a general anaesthetic without intubation.
- The child will be lying supine on the operating table.
- A basic set of instruments will be used.
- The child's head will be placed in a head ring.

PAEDIATRIC EYE SURGERY

Visual impairments are common in childhood, and the rate of children wearing glasses can be up to 3.5%, but only 0.5/1000 of those children will be legally blind.[7] Good vision is vitally important for learning and development, and refractive errors are the most common types of paediatric visual disorders. These often require surgical correction. Only a small number of paediatric ophthalmic surgery procedures are outlined here.

Nasolacrimal duct obstruction

Six per cent of infants have obstruction of their nasolacrimal duct, and 90% of these will clear spontaneously.[78] In babies less than 6 months of age, massage of the duct may clear it, and parents can be taught to do this once a day. If this fails, probing is required. A fine dilator is passed down the duct under general anaesthetic and the duct irrigated. In rare cases, probing has to be repeated.

Perioperative nursing implications

- The child will receive a general anaesthetic without intubation.
- The child will be lying supine on the operating table.
- A set of lacrimal probes will be used to probe the tear duct.
- The child's head will be placed in a head ring.

Squint repair

Strabismus is a visual defect in which the extraocular muscles cannot coordinate and direct the eyes in the same direction.[79] It affects up to 4% of children in some countries.[80] Occlusive therapy to strengthen the eye muscles may be tried, but often surgery is required.[7] The operative procedure to correct strabismus will depend on the muscles affected and which way the eye turns. Some muscles are shortened by resection, while others can be severed from their original attachment and replaced on a different position of the sclera to pull the eye in the required position (recession).[79,80]

Perioperative nursing implications

- The child will receive a general anaesthetic.
- The child will be lying supine on the operating table.
- A basic set of instruments will be used including squint repair instrumentation such as princess clamps to hold eye muscles and eyelid retractors.
- The child's head will be placed in a head ring.

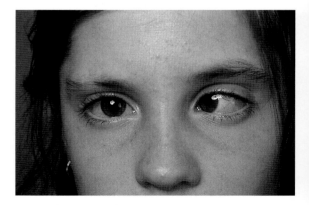

Fig. 10.19 Strabismus

- Bipolar diathermy will be used; therefore, no patient electrode/diathermy plate will be needed.
- Very small sutures will be used so special care with the fine needles must be taken.

PAEDIATRIC NEUROSURGERY

Ann Tanner

Paediatric neurosurgery has changed dramatically since the use of car seat belts has become widely accepted and the incidence of severe head injury has reduced, and with the successful treatment of conditions such as hydrocephalus.

Hydrocephalus

Hydrocephalus, or 'water on the brain', occurs when there is an increase of cerebrospinal fluid (CSF) in the brain and spinal cord because of obstruction, excessive production of CSF or under-absorption. It is often associated with myelomeningocele.[7] It was once a relatively common condition in infancy and very visible because of the deformity of the head which kept growing as fluid built up, eventually killing the child. With screening procedures in child health such as routine head circumference measurement, hydrocephalus is found and treated with insertion of a shunt to carry the excess fluid into a

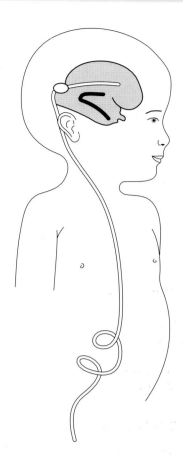

Fig. 10.21 Hydrocephalus: ventriculoperitoneal shunt

vein or the abdominal cavity. Hydrocephalus is still seen in developing countries where screening may not be available in remote villages.[81]

Surgical treatment involves the removal of the cause of the obstruction (e.g. a tumour) or the insertion of a shunt mechanism that allows excess CSF to flow away.[7] Most shunts consist of a catheter placed in the ventricles, a flush pump, a one-way valve and a distal catheter, which is placed in the peritoneum, or a cardiac atrium.[13] Shunts must be changed as the child grows.

A new technique – third ventriculostomy – has been developed for use in children with hydrocephalus caused by obstruction. Endoscopically, the surgeon punctures a hole between the subarachnoid space and the third ventricle creating a drainage pathway for the CSF.[82]

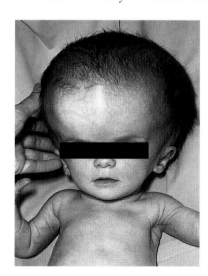

Fig. 10.20 Hydrocephalus: infant with untreated hydrocephalus

Craniotomy

Craniotomies are performed for a variety of reasons ranging from traumatic and closed head injuries to brain tumours, aneurysms and craniofacial surgery. A craniotomy involves the removal of a section of the skull, also known as a flap. Depending on the site of the craniotomy, the child may be positioned prone or supine. In the case of a brain tumour, the operation may take many hours to complete. Therefore, correct and safe patient positioning is required. This includes centering the patient on the bed, padding bony prominences, supporting limbs and using positioning devices where needed.[83]

Many surgical procedures involving the brain have an increased risk of morbidity or mortality. For the perioperative nurse scrubbing or scouting for the craniotomy, it is important to be prepared and commence setting up for the case as early as possible. In the larger booked cases, the anaesthetic preparation is much more involved. The patient will have a number of intravenous access lines and often will require an arterial line.[84] The airway is secured with occlusive and waterproof tapes. The eyes are protected with lubricant and covered by gauze and occlusive waterproof dressings. The patient may require a urinary catheter to monitor output, and may have a rectally inserted temperature probe. For the emergency admissions such as sub- and extradural haematomas, the child may arrive via computerised axial tomography (CAT) scan already intubated. This means that for the OR nurse, there is less set-up time, so speed and organisation are essential.

For the craniotomy, a neurosurgical headrest is often used, commonly the Mayfield headrest,[84] which consists of a head clamp in which three sterile pins are placed to pierce the scalp. The clamp is fixed to the head of the bed and immobilises the skull for surgery. The surgeon shaves the area of the head and marks the incision line with a permanent marker. The scrub nurse can then commence the skin preparation. A large semicircular incision is made into the scalp, and plastic skin clips (Leroy clips) are applied to the skin edges to maintain haemostasis as the skin over the skull is highly vascularised. A periosteal elevator is used to separate muscle from bone on the skull. The bone flap is removed using a powered drilling burr to make the initial hole in the skull, followed by a cutting drill bit, which cuts the bone in the same fashion as a jig saw. (The removed piece of bone is plated or wired back onto the skull following the surgery.) The exposed dura can then be picked up with a dural hook and an incision made into it with a clean blade followed by dissection with scissors. The dura is retracted with stay sutures, leaving the brain exposed for surgery.

Emergency craniotomies can be performed in the case of subdural and extradural haematomas. These can occur following a substantial blow to the skull where venous or arterial vessels are disrupted and bleed.[85] In the case of extradural haematomas, the bleed occurs between the skull and the dural space. These are more commonly arterial bleeds and, due to the rapidity of the bleed, are acute and life threatening, especially in children, if not surgically evacuated and the haemostasis controlled. The subdural bleeds are venous bleeds that occur between the brain and the dura. The surgical removal and control of subdural haematomas is the primary treatment of the brain injury; the ensuing intracranial hypertension from the trauma often indicates if and how well the patient will recover. The injury caused to the brain tends to be more severe for sub- than for extradural haematomas, and recovery is related to clinical presentation on arrival, including level of consciousness and pupillary reactions. The lower the neurological status on admission, the poorer the expected outcome to the surgery.

Perioperative nursing implications

There are a number of important issues to consider for the paediatric perioperative nurse. Organisation and preparation of the required equipment is essential. In the case of booked admissions, the child and their family may be extremely anxious before surgery. Older children with a greater understanding of the procedure may have received a premedication before admission to theatre to assist in the relief of anxiety. On admission to theatre, the perioperative nurse can help allay anxiety by introducing themselves to the child and their family, establishing a rapport with the parents. It is important that the OR staff have a contact number for the parents or have instructed them about where they can wait whilst their child undergoes surgery so that they are easily contacted should the surgeon need to speak to them during or after the procedure.

Spina bifida

Spina bifida is a congenital defect in which the neural tube has failed to close and is not fully encased in the protective sheath of the meninges and spine. The failure of the neural tube closure occurs early in the development of the embryo,[7] and this has been related to a deficiency of folate in early pregnancy.[86,87] In a normal spine, the spinal cord is in the spinal canal. It is an extension of the brain stem, commences in the first cervical vertebra (C1) and finishes at the second lumbar vertebra (L2). The lumbar spine encapsulates a vertical bundle of spinal nerves known as the *cauda equina*.[84] Spina bifida usually occurs in the lumbar or lumbar sacral region of the spine. The aetiology has been linked to an abnormal increase in CSF pressure during the first trimester of pregnancy causing a split in the previously enclosed neural tube. Hydrocephalus is commonly associated with spina bifida.[7]

There are varying degrees of severity of spina bifida. The mildest form is spina bifida occulta, where there is a gap in the vertebrae usually at the second lumbar vertebra, with no herniation of meninges or spinal cord and limited loss of sensation or function. Meningoceles occur when the meninges have herniated out of the gap in the vertebrae without involving the spinal cord. The herniated meninges form a cyst-like sack filled with the CSF.[7]

Children born with meningoceles can have varying degrees of sensory and motor impairment. Some may walk, but they have impairment or paralysis to the bladder and anal sphincter.

The most severe form of spina bifida is the myelomeningocele (sometimes called meningomyelocele). The meninges herniate out through the bony defect taking with them a portion of the spinal cord and nerves. These children can have full paralysis and complete sensory deficit below the region of the herniation.[7]

Surgical treatment of both the meningocele and the myelomeningocele involves initial closure of the herniated meninges and spinal cord. Surgical closure reduces the risk of infection. The procedure often requires a multidisciplinary approach involving a combination of neuro- and plastic surgeons. Children suffering from spina bifida often require multiple operations over many years. These range from ventriculoperitoneal shunts for congenital hydrocephalus to the creation of stomas for the bladder and bowel so that the child may self-catheterise via the abdomen, and may perform bowel washouts to prevent continuing incontinence. Some may need to undergo surgery for the placement of spinal rods or fusions to reduce curvature of the spine.

Perioperative nursing implications

It is important for the perioperative nurse to note that spina bifida children have a high incidence of latex allergies.[88] This is possibly as a result of their high exposure to latex products with their daily

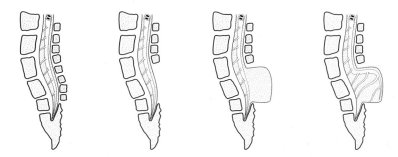

Fig. 10.22 Spina bifida: 1, normal spine; 2, spina bifida occulta; 3, spina bifida with meningocele; 4, spina bifida with myelomeningocele

Surgical procedures on children

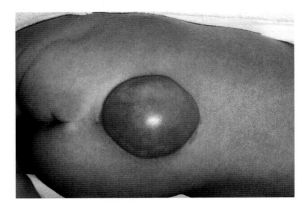

Fig. 10.23 Spina bifida: meningocele

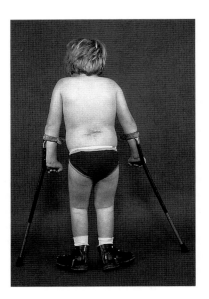

Fig. 10.25 Spina bifida: repair site and impairment of the lower back and legs

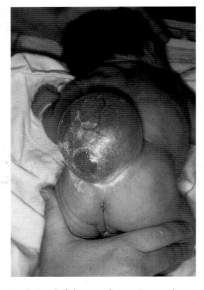

Fig. 10.24 Spina bifida: myelomeningocele

intermittent urinary catheterisations, and their frequent hospital admissions and subsequent exposure to the latex in the gloves worn by staff. It is important for the perioperative nurse to be aware of latex allergies, for at worst they can result in anaphylaxis (see Chapter 3).

PAEDIATRIC ORTHOPAEDICS

Orthopaedic surgery inovlves the skeletal system which includes bones, joints, muscles, tendons, ligaments and cartilage. Children require orthopaedic surgery for the correction of congenital deformities, washout of infections of the bone or joints, for removal of bone tumours and for the repair of injured or fractured limbs, joints, tendons or nerves as a result of trauma.

Perioperative nursing implications

For the perioperative nurse there are a number of common factors involved. Orthopaedics generally involves a limb as spinal and neck surgery is considered a subspecialty of orthopaedics. The limb is fully prepared and draped with extra waterproof mackintosh drapes and extra small and medium drapes to ensure blood or fluids do not penetrate the drapes and risk contaminating the wound. In many instances (except in trauma cases) a tourniquet is applied to the limb to block the arterial blood supply so that the procedure can be carried out in a bloodless field.[89] The tourniquet may remain on for up to 2 hours. It is important that the tourniquet cuff does not pinch the skin or the skin preparation fluid does not run under the cuff as both can cause significant burns to the child.[89]

Orthopaedic surgery often requires the use of a number of powered instruments. For those not familiar with power tools, their use requires a thorough 'hands on' education session. There is a whole range of nitrous cylinder-powered drills, taps, screws, burrs and saws to master for the perioperative nurse scrubbing for an orthopaedic case. An important point to remember is always to have the safety switch on when loading and unloading bone-cutting instruments.

Infection of bone or joint

When a child presents with acute commencement of pain, swelling or tenderness of any joint or limb, with an associated unwillingness to weight bear, the suspected prognosis is of osteomyelitis or septic arthritis.[90] The surgical treatment for such infections involves opening the infected section of the limb or joint and washing out the infected area. The child is routinely given antibiotic coverage during the procedure, and a specimen of pus is taken to determine the most effective course of antibiotics and the nature of the infection.

Congenital deformities

There are many differing congenital abnormalities that may benefit from surgical orthopaedic intervention. Talipes, or 'club feet', can be repaired by tendon release and transfers and a succession of plaster casts changed every 1–2 weeks to improve positioning.[90]

Children with cerebral palsy often require tendon release surgery and splinting to assist in gait and stance. Children born with shortened, stunted limbs, fused joints, extra or missing digits, missing bones, fragile bones (osteogenesis imperfecta), bowed legs, deformed feet and hands and many more are all potential candidates for corrective orthopaedic surgery.[90]

Bone tumours

Malignant bone tumours are more common in children than in adults, and the annual incidence is approximately 5.6 per million in children under 15 years of age.[91] The age group most at risk are the 15–19 year olds. This is thought to be related to the increased rate of bone tissue growth during that

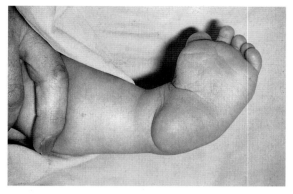

Fig. 10.26 Talipes: infant with 'club feet' – talipes

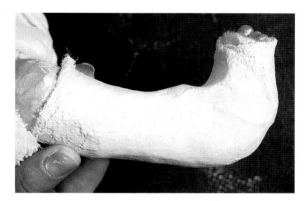

Fig. 10.27 Talipes: treated talipes in a plaster cast following remedial surgery

age. The two major types of bone tumours that make up 85% of cases are Ewing's sarcoma and osteogenic sarcoma.[7] Some of the clinical signs of a bone tumour are localised pain at the affected site, limping and generally limited activity. Occasionally the child may present with a pathological fracture as the first indication of a tumour. Bone tumours are primarily suspected whenever there is a fracture following a trivial fall.[90] Surgery is the primary method of treatment for a bone tumour. With increased technology, the limb can often be saved following excision of the affected bone (e.g. the femur) by means of a femoral prosthesis. Before such advances in prosthetic surgery, the limb would have been amputated.

Fractures in children

Owing to children's natural curiosity and play behaviour, they are much more physically active than adults and have a greater risk of falls and limb fractures. The causes of such fractures include falls from playground equipment, trampolines, bicycles, roller blades, skate boards, scooters, trees, etc. Fractures in children differ from adults in that the growing child is at risk of growth plate injuries that can stunt the growth of the affected limb. One-third of fractures suffered by children involve the growth plate.[90]

A commonly found fracture in children is a metaphyseal fracture to the distal radius, ulna or tibia. There are three types: 1, buckle fracture, where the compressed metaphyseal bone elevates the cortical surface of the bone, giving a buckled appearance; 2, greenstick fracture, an incomplete break where one side of the cortex is compressed and remains intact while the other side breaks, causing the bone to angulate; and 3, a complete fracture, which can be displaced or undisplaced, and in severe trauma may be compound, where the fracture protrudes from the skin.[90]

Treatment of fractures in children ranges from a closed reduction under a general anaesthetic, where the surgeon manipulates the fracture and provides traction on the limb until the bone is realigned. In more severe fractures, the child may require an open reduction and internal fixation of the fracture. The fixation can be in the form of wires, plates and screws.

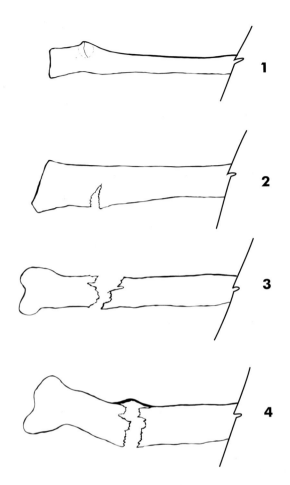

Fig. 10.28 Common fractures in children: 1 buckle fracture, 2 greenstick fracture, 3 complete fracture, 4 periosteal hinge

Congenital hip dysplasia

Congenital hip dysplasia is more commonly known as developmental dysplasia of the hip, as it is now recognised that at birth, the hips are rarely dislocated but are easily 'dislocatable'.[92] This is recognised soon after birth by routine examination of the hips and is often treated conservatively with traction and splints.[7] In older infants and more severe cases, surgical treatment to reposition the joint may be needed.[92]

PAEDIATRIC PLASTIC SURGERY

Paediatric plastic surgery involves the surgical reconstruction and repair of congenital abnormalities, injury (e.g. facial fractures), disfigurement and scarring. Plastic surgery is the process of restoring the normal appearance and of achieving normal function where possible.[93] Some of the more common plastics procedures performed on children are outlined below.

Craniofal surgery

Craniofacial surgery involves a team of plastic surgeons and neurosurgeons. The plastic surgery team is responsible for the remodelling of facial and cranial bones and structures; the neurosurgeon performs the craniotomy (see 'Craniotomy'). The child may require craniofacial surgery because of premature fusion of the cranial sutures of the skull that need to be released and remoulded.[94] There may be an encephalocele,[95] a sac-like extrusion as a result of some form of facial cleft, usually from the midline of the nose, that can contain CSF and brain tissue, or may be independent of the brain. If there is neurological involvement, it can take many hours to excise surgically and to realign the facial cleft.

Cleft lip and palate repair

Cleft lip and palate are congenital abnormalities that can occur in 1:750–2500 live births, and are more common in males.[96] They are facial malformations that occur during the development of the embryo, and while no one cause is known, inheritance,[97] ethnicity and maternal drug exposure are thought to play a part. A cleft lip is the failure of the maxillary and median processes to fuse; a cleft palate is a failure of fusion of the midline of the palate resulting in a fissure in it.[7] Cleft lips can occur uni- or bilaterally and can occur in conjunction with a cleft palate. Usually, the more severe bilateral cleft lips occur with a cleft palate.

The surgical treatment involves the repair of the cleft lip at about 3 months of age when it is believed the infant has sufficient weight gain and lung function to withstand a general anaesthetic. The cleft palate is often repaired in two stages, initially with the hard palate repair followed by the soft palate repair, although other techniques are commonly used.[98] The severity of the cleft determines the amount of surgery required. The primary palate repair is usually performed at 6 months of age, with the secondary repair at 9 or 10 months of age. Many surgeons like to repair the palate before the child develops faulty speech patterns.[7]

Setback otoplasty

A setback otoplasty is commonly referred to as correction of protruding ears and is most often done for cosmetic reasons, as these children often become victims of mockery and abuse by their peers.[99] Otoplasty often involves an incision to the back of the ear and the ear is resected down to the cartilage layer, the cartilage scored with a blade or a specially

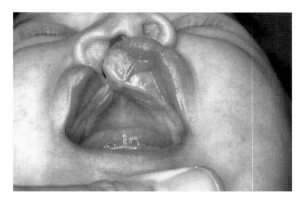

Fig. 10.29 Cleft lip and palate

designed raked forceps so that it can be reshaped and moulded closer to the head.[100] The incision is closed and a head bundle dressing applied, which remains intact until follow-up review, usually 10 days after surgery, though some surgeons require the bandages to remain on for much shorter periods.[101] The moulding created by the head bundle helps the ears to sit closer to the head as the wound heals. Some postoperative considerations include the fact that the child has a complete head bundle dressing occluding the ears and can be slightly deaf, may suffer nausea and may need antiemetics.

Hand and foot deformities

There are many deformities of the hands and feet that require plastic surgery intervention. In basic terms, syndactyly occurs when the digits are joined by a web of skin, can be complete or incomplete, depending on the number of digits involved, and can be complex or simple, depending on the level of bony union between the involved digits. Polydactyly is the duplication of some digits and can be simple or complex depending on bony involvement.[102] In surgery for syndactyly, the digits are separated by a series of z-plasties, zigzag incisions to divide the joined digits. These are resutured and each digit wrapped in a supportive dressing. The dressing forms an integral part of the repair as it helps to shape and mould the digit as the wound heals and acts in a splinting capacity. Surgery for polydactyly can be a simple removal of extra digits, or very

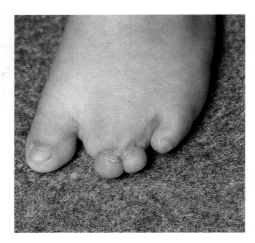

Fig. 10.30 Hand and foot deformities: syndactyly of the foot

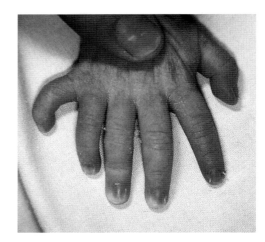

Fig. 10.32 Hand and foot deformities: polydactyly of the hand

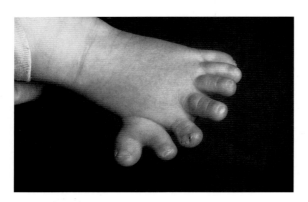

Fig. 10.31 Hand and foot deformities: polydactyly of the foot

complex reconstruction of the whole hand. This type of plastic surgery can be very involved and take several hours to complete, especially if both hands/feet are affected.

Skin lesions

There are many types of skin lesions that can require plastic surgical intervention. Some of the most common are outlined below.

Dermoid cysts are congenital cysts. They are usually rounded, soft and often fixed to deep tissues or bone. In children, they are commonly found under the lateral part of the eyebrow, the scalp, the tip of the nose and the orbit.[103] Naevus is a term applied to 'any skin lesion appearing at or after birth'[104] (p. 955) and covers a wide range of conditions, from the trivial to melanoma, which may have the potential to become malignant (metastatic melanoma). They can be non-melanocytic, in which case there is very little risk of malignancy and little need for excision unless the naevus is disfiguring. The naevus can range in size, pigmentation, colour and appear with or without hair, occasionally having a velvet texture.[104] Treatment for the melanocytic naevus usually involves surgical excision, with the specimen sent to pathology. This is particularly the case if there is a family history of malignant melanoma.

Haemangiomas[105] are the most common tumours in infants and cover a wide complex of conditions from simple 'birth marks' to involvement of complex arterial systems and various organs. They are vascular in nature; some resolve spontaneously, some respond to treatments such as compression, radiation, steroids and sclerotherapy. Some haemangiomas can be fatal, especially if they occlude vital organs. Surgical intervention is governed by the position, size and organ involvement and can include excision by conventional methods and laser.

Childhood burns

Childhood burns are potentially one of the most disfiguring injuries that can occur to a child. They

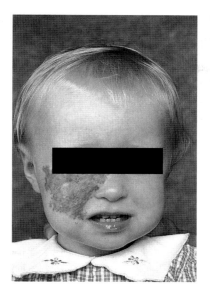

Fig. 10.33 Skin lesion: a child with facial haemangioma

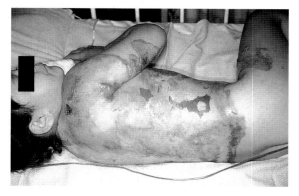

Fig. 10.34 Burns: a child with severe burns

can require long-term hospital intervention, including surgery and follow-up scar management, including the use of pressure garments and intensive physiotherapy and occupational therapy. The trauma involved for the child and their family is immense and even after aggressive surgical intervention they can still be left with life-long horrific disfigurements. The most common type of childhood burn results from scald burns[106–108] from incidents including pulling saucepans of hot liquids off stoves, tea or coffee spills, and bath or hot tap water burns.[109]

Scalds play such an important role in paediatric thermal injuries because many households have their hot water systems set as high as 70°C, at which it takes one-quarter of a second for a child to sustain a full-thickness, third-degree burn requiring skin grafting and scar management. At 60°C, it takes 1 second for the child to sustain full-thickness burns; at 55°C, it takes 10 seconds and at 50°C, it takes 5 minutes to sustain full-thickness burns.[110]

Although scald burns account for only a small proportion of hospital admissions for childhood injuries, they are one of the three leading causes of hospital admission amongst children.[111] The treatment of burns is extremely costly, particularly when the burn is a full thickness (third degree), where

permanent and often disfiguring scarring results with the need for skin-grafting and use of pressure garments.

Following a major burn, there is a large movement of fluids from the vascular compartments to the interstitial spaces, most dramatically in the first 6–12 hours. The capillaries' permeability is rapidly altered following a burn injury allowing plasma, proteins, water and electrolytes to leak into the interstitial spaces of both injured and non-injured tissue. The greatest amount of swelling occurs in the first 36 hours postburn; hence, the 36 hours standard fluid resuscitation period. Following the initial resuscitation period, there continues to be a large amount of leakage of water, sodium and plasma from the open burn throughout the recovery period until the burn injury is covered by means of surgical skin grafting.[112] Resuscitation fluids and a catheter are required for any baby (0–12 months) whose burns are > 10% or any child whose burns are > 15% (excluding erythema).

For full-thickness and some partial-thickness burns, the surgical treatment is early excision and grafting.[113] A full-thickness burn should be excised and grafted as soon as the patient is haemodynamically stable, usually after the first 36 hours of fluid resuscitation. This early excision and grafting has been shown to reduce the length of hospital stay. With the surgical excision of burns, most wounds can be immediately grafted. The harvested skin is usually partial thickness, which reduces scarring to the donor site and effectively covers the area of excised skin. Burns surgery can result in a large blood and fluid loss. Perioperative nursing considerations include maintaining a warm room temperature, as the blood and fluid loss has a concomitant loss of body temperature. The need for complete sterility cannot be stressed enough: infected graft sites do not take and can lead to increased scarring.

PAEDIATRIC UROLOGY

Urology encompasses diseases and malformation of the adrenal glands, kidneys, ureter, bladder, female and male genitalia, including for the male the penis, urethra, prostate gland and scrotum. Some of the more common procedures in paediatric urology are outlined below.

Cystoscopy and urethroscopy

Cystoscopy and urethroscopy involve inserting a scope into the bladder and urethra respectively.[114] In children these procedures are usually performed under a general anaesthetic. The child's legs will be placed in stirrups so that the urethra is easily accessed. The perianal area is prepared, and a window sheet used as a drape, along with small drapes to cover the child's legs. The scope has a telescope, light source and irrigation line attached. The telescope may or may not be connected to a television monitor. In children, the urethral valves may need dissecting, and the surgeon may use a paediatric resectoscope, and may diathermy the urethral obstruction.[115] The child needs a diathermy plate for this procedure. Because the diathermy is performed in a liquid field, the irrigation solution used must be non-conductive to prevent burns. Usually glycine 1.5% solution is used. For all other cysto- and urethroscopies not involving diathermy, normal saline is used for irrigation.

Ureteropelvic junction (UPJ) obstruction

A UPJ obstruction occurs when there is insufficient drainage of urine from the renal pelvis into the upper ureter. This can result in distension of the renal pelvis, raised intrapelvic pressure and kidney damage from the stasis of urine in the collecting ducts.[116] UPJ obstruction results from a narrowing of the ureteropelvic junction, which may form a partial or complete obstruction. The surgical treatment is by means of a pyeloplasty in which the renal pelvis is reduced, the ureter divided below the obstruction, then reanastomosed to the renal pelvis above the site of the obstruction.

Ureteric reimplantation

Ureteric reimplants are indicated when the ureters are significantly dilated, often termed 'mega-ureter'.[116] The ureter can be refluxing, obstructed, non-refluxing or non-obstructed. The reflux can be congenital or as a result of the urethral valves or a neurogenic bladder. The obstruction may be primary (adynamic segment) or secondary to an urethral obstruction, mass or tumour. Ureteric reimplants can be unilateral or bilateral. For the procedure, a longitudinal segment of the ureter is excised and closed over a 10- or 12-French catheter; the ureter is then tunnelled submucosally into the bladder. There is an 85–95% success rate for a non-refluxing, non-obstructive reimplantation.[116]

ANAESTHESIA OF CHILDREN

Annabel Herron and Linda Shields

Anaesthetics delivered to children differ greatly from those used on adult patients for many reasons. Differences in size, immaturity of organ systems and, most importantly, the child's psychological development are important factors in paediatric anaesthesia. General anaesthetics are often given to children for procedures that might normally not require an anaesthetic or could be controlled by a local anaesthetic in an adult. Children often cannot cope physiologically and psychologically with unfamiliar environments, parental separation and/or minimal pain. For a full description of the role of the anaesthetic nurse, see Chapter 7. In this section, paediatric anaesthesia is briefly discussed.

Temperature regulation is of utmost importance in paediatric anaesthetics. The small size, increased body surface area:body weight ratio and increased heat conductivity contribute to anaesthetic risk in infants and small children.[117] Consequently, the use of warming equipment during anaesthesia is always a consideration in paediatrics. Such equipment includes anaesthetic gas warmers, IV warmers and warming blankets for underneath and on top of the patient. ORs and units should also have OR temperature regulators that can be changed to suit the environment required for the child.

Blood conservation is also an important factor in paediatric anaesthesia.[118] Because of children's size and weight, they have a smaller blood volume than an adult. Therefore, the anaesthetist will constantly consider the amount of blood lost intraoperatively and endeavour to replace it. It is important for the perioperative nurse to keep the anaesthetist updated by checking and recording blood lost from the suction and swabs by measuring and weighing all articles containing blood. Particular care must be taken to ensure these weights are accurate as it is very easy, and dangerous, to over-transfuse an infant.

TYPES OF ANAESTHETICS

Topical anaesthetic creams that anaesthetise a small area of skin and make IV access painless have revolutionised paediatric anaesthesia. These creams are developing, but one of the most commonly used is EMLA™ cream, which is composed of lignocaine and prilocaine.[119] It numbs the skin by releasing these agents into the epidermal and dermal layers, making IV line insertion painless, and thereby reduces the psychological stress endured by the child. IV agents used to induce anaesthesia can then be administered to the child with minimal discomfort.

General anaesthesia (GA)

'General anaesthesia is a reversible, unconscious state characterised by amnesia (sleep, hypnosis, or basal narcosis), analgesia (freedom from pain), depression of reflexes, muscle relaxation, and haemostasis or specific manipulation of physiological systems and function'[5] (p. 208). GA is commonly used in paediatrics as children are less likely to cope psychologically with being awake for operative procedures, and many minor procedures are done using GA.

Perioperative nursing considerations

Recording the child's height and weight is important as these parameters are required for temperature control, calculation of blood loss, anaesthetic

induction and agents and maintenance equipment. Intubation equipment such as laryngoscope blades, endotracheal tubes (ETTs), laryngeal mask airways (LMAs) and guedel airways must be size-appropriate for the age and weight of the child. Electrocardiograph (ECG) monitoring 'dots' are size specific and should fit the child appropriately and not occlude the surgical field.

Regional anaesthesia

Regional anaesthesia is broadly defined as 'a reversible loss of sensation in a specific area or region of the body when local anaesthetic is injected to purposefully block or anaesthetise nerve fibres in and around the operative site'[5] (p. 208). Common regional anaesthesia techniques include spinal, epidural, caudal and major peripheral nerve blocks.

Caudal analgesia is probably the most useful and popular paediatric regional block used, especially in procedures in areas below the umbilicus.[120] A needle is inserted into the caudal space in the lower spine and drugs (the dose calculated on the weight of the child) injected. The most common drug used is bupivicaine. Duration of a caudal block is usually about 2–4 hours, depending on the strength of the drug. Complications can include ineffectiveness (the block does not work) and inadvertent intravenous injection. It is considered a reliable, safe and easy to perform procedure in children, especially in patients weighing > 10 kg.[117]

Epidural anaesthesia is becoming accepted in paediatric anaesthesia, though it is still not as commonly used as caudal block. Both intermittent and continuous epidural blockade for infants and children undergoing orthopaedic, abdominal and thoracic surgery have been used.[117] Epidural blocks are not used alone in children, rather they are supplemented with light general anaesthesia.[120]

Spinal anaesthetics are used generally on the premature neonate at risk of postoperative apnoea which is common after a general anaesthetic in ventilated infants.[117] They are rarely used on other children because of the loss of motor power which can distress and frighten children.[120]

Perioperative nursing considerations

Equipment used to induce regional anaesthetics must be considered when preparing for the procedure. Epidural and spinal kits that are size appropriate to the child must be available. Consider also the patient's positioning, either lying laterally with the knees bent towards the chest; sitting upright, curved over, with their chin towards their chest; or as the anaesthetist desires. Spinal anaesthetics on neonates and infants are usually performed with an awake child, so the child must be held tightly to prevent excessive movements or squirming. This can be distressing for the child, the parents and for staff. Support must be provided for all and explanation of the procedure, its rationale and implementation provided at all times.

Conscious sedation/anaesthesia

Conscious sedation can be described as 'a state that allows patients to tolerate unpleasant procedures while maintaining adequate cardiorespiratory function and the ability to respond purposefully to verbal command and/or tactile stimulation'[5] (p. 208). This type of anaesthetic is rarely used in paediatrics except in adolescents having a minor procedure, e.g. endoscopy or insertion of an IV access device. The procedure must be discussed with the child and his/her informed consent obtained before administration.

Perioperative nursing considerations

If the adolescent requires conscious sedation, the perioperative nurse should consider that the patient is in a state of consciousness and give explanations and reassurance at all times. Parents must be kept fully informed and allowed to participate (in both the procedure and decision-making about it) as required by them and the child. Equipment necessary for anaesthetic administration should be available to the anaesthetist at all times.

Local anaesthesia

Local anaesthesia refers to the 'administration of an anaesthetic agent to one part of the body by local infiltration or topical application'[5] (p. 209). It is used widely in paediatrics as a method of postoperative pain relief. Dosages of local anaesthetics in children are based on a dose per weight calculation and these must be strictly adhered to. Overdoses and toxicity

are easy when doses and amounts are very small. Often, agents such as bupivicaine are infiltrated into operation sites at the end of an operation to provide initial pain relief.[120] Often, by the time the local analgesia effect has worn off, the child will require little more than paracetamol for postoperative pain relief.

Perioperative nursing considerations

Dosages are calculated on the weight of the child. At present, recommendations for maximum safe doses of local anaesthetic agents are based largely on data obtained in adults and a dose per weight calculation,[117] so the scrub nurse must always double check the amount and strength of the required drug with the anaesthetist or surgeon before drawing the drug into the syringe before administration. When applying EMLA cream, the perioperative nurse must consider whether the child will tamper with the cream and the occlusive dressing and remove it. If they believe it is a possibility, then measures must be taken to prevent it, such as securely bandaging the extremity and explaining to the parent the importance of leaving the dressing in place for at least 30 minutes before IV insertion.

PAEDIATRIC POSTANAESTHETIC RECOVERY

Lee-Anne Waterman

The perioperative nurse in the Paediatric Post-Anaesthesia Care Unit (PPACU) is an integral member of the operating team who cares for the patient during the immediate postanaesthetic phase of surgical or procedural intervention. They assess, plan, deliver and evaluate the care of the paediatric surgical patient and act as advocate for the child promoting physical, psychological, and spiritual wellbeing and safety.

All children who have a general or local anaesthetic are cared for postoperatively in the PPACU. The length of stay there depends on the condition of the patient and the surgical procedure. Close observation is vital during this phase as consciousness and reflexes may still be impaired. It is important to recognise that children are different to adults physiologically, psychologically and emotionally, and their care while in the PPACU must reflect this.

PPACUs should be near the ORs to ensure that the patient can be returned immediately to surgery if needed or so that OR staff can attend quickly. The unit itself is an 'open ward' design to facilitate observation of all patients simultaneously. The room in general and each patient space should be well lit and large enough for easy access to the child in spite of IV equipment, monitoring equipment, heaters or ventilation equipment. Each bed space should be equipped with an oxygen, air and suction outlet as well as with multiple electrical outlets.[121]

Table 10.1
Initial assessment of a child on entry to the PPACU
■ Skin colour: cyanosis and/or shock ■ Respirations: rate, depth and sounds ■ Temperature: hypothermic: hyperthermic perfusion ■ Blood pressure and pulse: rate, volume, rhythm ■ Level of consciousness: reflexes (cough, swallow), rousability ■ Wounds and drains: haemorrhage

Standards of care

The first and most important responsibility of the registered nurse (RN) in the PPACU is to the child, and the RN must be present at all times when a patient is in the room. All postanaesthetic nursing care of children should be managed by appropriately trained and qualified postanaesthetic care RNs, though this is often difficult. There should be a 1:1 nurse to patient ratio in unrousable patients.[122] Children respond to anaesthetic and its subsequent reversal very quickly. The anaesthetic process by its nature is experienced by a child as a time when they are in a strange environment surrounded by people they do not know where they cannot stay with their parents. Depending on the nature of the surgery (elective or emergency; major or minor, the preparation the child has received and their cognitive abilities), the child in the PPACU has to be viewed as fully dependent, and it is the RN's responsibility to prevent injury and reduce distress as much as possible.

Routine recovery

Initial phase

Patients should not leave the OR unless they have a stable and patent airway, have adequate ventilation and oxygenation, and are haemodynamically stable. Transporting the child from the OR to the PPACU, the child should be positioned on their side (lateral) to prevent complications from vomiting or postoperative bleeding, and on a bed that can be placed head up or down (Trendelenburg position). The down position is used for children with hypovolaemia and the up position for children with underlying respiratory prob-

lems such as asthma or cystic fibrosis. The bed should have oxygen, mask, T-piece and a bag available.

On arrival in the PPACU, initial observations are commenced immediately. The child's airway must be patent with adequate ventilation and oxygen should be administered as soon as possible. Often the child will have an airway such as guedel or LMA *in situ*. Oxygen saturation with pulse monitoring should commence and the child's respirations be checked for rate, depth and sounds. The child's colour and rousability should be assessed.

Continuous observation of the child while receiving a handover from the anaesthetist is vital. The immediate PPACU period is the most dangerous and the most common serious problems are related to airway obstruction and respiratory depression. While noisy breathing is always obstructed breathing, obstructed breathing is not always noisy. It is extremely important that the RN is positioned so that the child can be seen and assessed continuously. This is usually at the head of the bed.

Ongoing phase

Following handover, observations should be noted every 5 minutes for at least 15 minutes or until stable, and every 15 minutes after that until discharge from the PPACU. Wounds and dressings should be checked for signs of ooze or haemorrhage and drain sites for leaking and patency. Routinely, blood pressure should be taken 15 minutely but more frequently if required. In cases of minor surgery, this may not be necessary and should be assessed individually. Temperature, especially in babies and neonates, should be checked continuously until stable and be within an acceptable range. Pain,

Table 10.2
Ongoing assessment

- Airway: position, obstruction, respirations, oxygen saturations
- Circulation: pulse, blood pressure, colour
- Temperature
- Consciousness: rousability, sedation
- Pain: including narcotic and epidural infusions
- Nausea and vomiting
- Wound ooze, drains, dressings
- IVT/epidural: patient, running
- Special observations as required: circulation observations for orthopaedic cases
- BSL as required

nausea and vomiting should be checked and assessed.

Infusions, IV bungs, drains and dressings once checked for patency and complications need to be checked for safety. Children, depending on age and stage, will often remove these in reaction to the fear and pain they may have experienced or be experiencing. IV lines should be secured with devices such as an armboard and bandage to prevent the child pulling them out or hurting itself with any of the device pieces. Infusions should always be connected to a volumetric infusion pump to ensure the child receives the fluid and to prevent fluid overload. Dressings and drains should be secured with appropriate tapes, bandages or splints so as not to compromise the wound or observations and to protect the wound for the child. Unlike adults, once the child is awake, it will be immediately mobile in most cases.

Observation and documentation

Accurate documentation of all fluids correctly being administered and intraoperative losses is very important. The younger the child, the more it is at risk. Children enter the OR in a fluid-depleted state after fasting for 4–6 hours. Their metabolic rate is twice that of an adult and they lose more water through evaporation than excretion. Renal function is immature, which limits the capacity to respond to fluid shifts and the ability to make urine.[123] Intraoperative fluid management considers maintenance requirements, preoperative deficit (duration of fasting), blood loss and third space loss.[121]

Pain and vomiting

Pain and vomiting are assessed and managed according to the anaesthetist's orders or the standing orders of the unit. In the early minutes of recovery, both acute pain and nausea can rouse children. Their responses can range from pale, clammy skin to tachycardia and pyrexia, to crying, screaming and thrashing around. The child is not yet fully conscious and they are often inconsolable, even in the company of their parents. Pain relief medication and antiemetics given promptly will prevent possible injury and stop the emotional trauma from escalating.

Special needs in the PPACU

The need to understand paediatric procedures is important. For example, in children having plastic surgery such as cleft palate and lip, not only do they have a seriously compromised airway including the possibility of obstruction or aspiration from ooze, but also this particular group of patients are babies who get basic comfort from sucking anything, e.g. soothers, fingers and teats, and will often try to. If

Table 10.3
Paediatric fluid-maintenance chart and formulas

Weight (kg)	24 h	Hourly (ml h^{-1})
Newborns	60–100 ml kg^{-1} / 24 h^{-1}	
0–10	100 ml kg^{-1} / 24 h^{-1}	4–40
11–20	1000 ml for the first 10 kg + 50 ml kg^{-1} for each kg over 10 kg	40–60
21–30	1500 ml for the first 20 kg + 25 ml kg^{-1} for each kg over 20 kg	60–70
31–60	1750 ml for the first 30 kg + 10 ml kg^{-1} for each kg over 30 kg	70–85

allowed, this can cause major damage to the repair. Preventing the sucking may also greatly distress children, and this can also cause an increase in wound ooze and damage to the repair. Therefore, these children need specially prepared arm splints and appro-

priate postoperative sedation. Other special needs include children who have diabetes, cystic fibrosis, birth defects, congenital syndromes, and respiratory, muscle and cardiac conditions.

Parents can be very helpful in the recovery phase, especially in cases where the child comes to the OR often, or has special needs such as deafness, blindness, language barriers, autism, etc. It is important, however, that the privacy and safety of the other patients, the child and the parents are considered. The PPACU is, by nature, a clinical unit, a closed environment, and an environment where many interventions may be happening at any given time to several patients. Some parents on entering a PPACU will feel faint and nauseous after a short time and there should always be sufficient staff to manage these situations should they arise. Parents need to be fully informed before their child's opera-

---

Table 10.4
Criteria for discharge from the PPACU

- Easily aroused
- Can maintain and protect the airway
- Stable vital signs approximate to normal preoperative values or within parameters laid down by the anaesthetist
- No obvious surgical complications
- Pain, nausea and vomiting are under control
- Appropriate documentation has been completed
- Child is clean, dry, warm and comfortable

Table 10.5
Developmental stages of children and perioperative nursing considerations

Age	Infant (birth to 11 months)	Toddler (1 to 3 years)	Preschool child (4 to 5 years)	School-age child (6 to 12 years)	Adolescent (13 to 18 years)
Stage	Bonded to parents/immediate family Sensitive to surroundings Very little language	More individual Assertive and willful Basic language	Fantasy and magical thinking Good language and cognition Strong sense of self	Well developed language with an ability to reason Early self control Basic idea of body functions Beginning concept of death	Independence Peer importance Realistic idea of death
Fears	Mistrust	Any parental separation Pain	Pain Disfigurement Frustration Long parental separation	Punishment of pain Disfigurement Death	Loss of autonomy Being trapped Peer pressure Death
Response	Stranger anxiety Crying Withdrawal	Tantrums and loss of control Hyperactive	Withdrawal Fantasy Anger	Withdrawal Demanding behaviour	Stubbornness Stoicism Depression Helplessness
Nursing	Enable parent involvement Provide a warm, caring environment and reduce extraneous noises and activity	Enable parent involvement Talk to the child Offer choices as much as possible	Enable parent involvement Talk to the child Use dolls to explain procedures and encourage fantasy or play	Respect the child's privacy. Talk with child, be positive about what will happen and encourage them to master the situation. Use dolls for explanations and play.	Orientate to and explain what is happening and why Encourage discussion about fears and concerns Enable control and choice Stress peer acceptance

tion and know that they need to be with their child as soon as possible on their waking postoperation. Depending on the policy of different hospitals, this may or may not occur in the PPACU. It is very important that nursing staff recognise when their paediatric patients are rousable and safe, and get them back to the postoperative care unit and their parents promptly.

Discharge

Criteria for discharge from the PPACU are established by the policy of the hospital and relevant anaesthetic department guidelines. Consequently, in many places, the RN determines when the child can be transferred providing all the criteria have been met.

References

1. Esposito C. One-trocar appendectomy in paediatric surgery. *Surg Endosc* 1998; 12: 177–178.
2. Luks FI, Logan J, Breuer CK, Kurkchubasche AG, Wessellhoeft CW, Tracy TF. Cost-effectiveness of laparoscopy in children. *Arch Pediatr Adolesc Med* 1999; 153: 965–968.
3. Ein SH. Appendicitis. In: Ashcraft KW, Murphy JP, Sharp RJ, Sigalet DL, Snyder CL. *Paediatric Surgery*, 3rd edn. Philadelphia: WB Saunders, 2000.
4. Anderson KN, Anderson LE, Glanze WD eds. *Mosby's Medical, Nursing and Allied Health Dictionary*, 4th edn. St Louis: Mosby, 1994.
5. Meeker RH, Rothrock JC. *Alexander's Care of the Patient in Surgery*, 11th edn. St Louis: Mosby, 1999.
6. Filston HC, Shorter NA. Esophageal atresia and tracheoesophageal malformations. In: Ashcraft KW, Murphy JP, Sharp RJ, Sigalet DL, Snyder CL. *Pediatric Surgery*, 3rd edn. Philadelphia: WB Saunders, 2000.
7. Whaley LF, Wong DL. *Whaley & Wong's Nursing Care of Infants and Children*, 5th edn. St Louis: Mosby 1995.
8. Games BA, Holcomb GW, Neblett WW. Gastroschisis and omphalocele. In: Ashcraft KW, Murphy JP, Sharp RJ, Sigalet DL, Snyder CL. *Pediatric Surgery*, 3rd edn. Philadelphia: WB Saunders, 2000.
9. Moushey R, Hawley C, Diomede B. Care of the pediatric patient. In: Phippen ML, Wells MP. *Patient Care during Operative and Invasive Procedures*. Philadelphia: WB Saunders, 2000.
10. Nuchtern JG, Baxter R, Hatch EL. Nonoperative initial management versus silon chimney for treatment of giant omphalocele. *J Paediatr Surg* 1995; 30: 771–776.
11. Hutson JM, Woodward AA, Beasley SW. *Jones' Clinical Paediatric Surgery: Diagnosis and Management*, 5th edn. Melbourne: Blackwell Science Asia, 1999.
12. Garcia VF. Umbilical and other abdominal wall hernias. In: Ashcraft KW, Murphy JP, Sharp RJ, Sigalet DL, Snyder CL. *Paediatric Surgery*, 3rd edn. Philadelphia: WB Saunders, 2000.
13. Maldonado S, Nygren C. Pediatric surgery. In: Meeker MH, Rothrock JC. *Alexander's Care of the Patient in Surgery*, 11th edn. Mosby: St Louis, 1999.
14. Fallat ME. Intussuseption. In: Asheraft KW, Murphy JP, Sharp RJ, Sigalet DL, Snyder CL. *Pediatric Surgery*, 3rd edn. Philadelphia: WB Saunders, 2000.
15. Chandler JH, Hebra A. Necrotizing enterocolitis in infants with very low birthweight. *Semin Pediatr Surg* 2000; 9: 63–72.
16. Caty MG, Azizkhan RG. Necrotizing enterocolitis. In: Ashcraft KW, Murphy JP, Sharp RJ, Sigalet DL, Snyder CL. *Pediatric Surgery*, 3rd edn. Philadelphia: WB Saunders, 2000.
17. Telemo E, Hansen LA. Antibodies in milk. *J Mammary Gland Biol Neoplasia* 1996; 1: 243–249.
18. Coit AK. Necrotizing enterocolitis. *J Perinat Neonatal Nurs* 1999; 12: 53–66.
19. Kennedy KA, Tyson JE, Chamnanvanakij S. Rapid versus slow rate of advancement of feelings for promoting growth and preventing necrotizing enterocolitis in parenterally fed low-birth-weight infants. *Cochrane Database Syst Rev* 2000; 2: CD001241.
20. Dillon PW, Cilley RE. Lesions of the stomach. In: Ashcraft KW, Murphy JP, Sharp RJ, Sigalet DL, Snyder CL. *Pediatric Surgery*, 3rd edn. Philadelphia: WB Saunders, 2000.
21. Bauchner H. Circumcision in the United States – the debate continues. *Arch Dis Child* 2000; 82: 357.
22. Goodman J. Circumcision is never right, be it male or female. *Nurs Times* 1998; 94.
23. Ponsky LE, Ross JH, Knipper N, Kay R. Penile adhesions after neonatal circumcision. *J Urol* 2000; 164: 495–496.
24. Williams CP, Richardson BG, Bukowski TP. Importance of identifying the inconspicuous penis: prevention of circumcision complications. *Urology* 2000; 56: 140–143.
25. Raynor SC. Circumcision. In: Ashcraft KW, Murphy JP, Sharp RJ, Sigalet DL, Snyder CL. *Paediatric Surgery*, 3rd edn. Philadelphia: WB Saunders, 2000.
26. Wallen EM, Shortliffe LMD. Undescended testis and testicular tumors. In: Ashcraft KW, Murphy JP, Sharp RJ, Sigalet DL, Snyder CL. *Paediatric Surgery*, 3rd edn. Philadelphia: WB Saunders, 2000.
27. Duckett JW. Hypospadias. *Pediatir Rev* 1989; 11: 37–42.
28. Silver RI. What is the etiology of hypospadias? A review of recent research. *Del Med J* 2000; 72: 343–347.
29. Safe SH. Endocrine disruptors and human health – is there a problem? An update. *Environ Health Perspec* 2000; 108: 487–493.
30. Landrigen PJ, Carlson, Bearer CF, Cranmer JS, Bullard RD, Etzel RA, Groopman J, McLachlan JA, Perera FP, Reigart JR, Robison L, Schell L, Suk WA. Children's

health and the environment: a new agenda for prevention research. *Environ Health Perspect* 1998; 106 (suppl.): 787–794.

31. Aho M, Koivisto AM, Tammela TL, Auvinen A. Is the incidence of hypospadias increasing? Analysis of Finnish hospital discharge 1970–1994. *Environ Health Perspec* 2000; 108: 463–465.

32. Chamber EL, Malone PS. The incidence of hypospadias in two English cities: a case-control comparison of possible causal factors. *Br J Urol Int* 1999; 84: 95–98.

33. Borer JG, Retik AB. Current trends in hypospadias repair. *Urol Clin North Am* 1999; 26: 15–37, vii.

34. Ellsworth P, Cendron M, Ritland D, McCullough M. Hypospadias repair in the 1990s. *AORN J* 1999; 69: 148–150, 152–153, 155–156.

35. Arensman RM, Bambini DA. Congenital diaphragmatic hernia and eventration. In: Ashcraft KW, Murphy JP, Sharp RJ, Sigalet DL, Snyder CL. *Paediatric Surgery*, 3rd edn. Philadelphia: WB Saunders, 2000.

36. Milwaukee Instate of' Minimally Invasive Surgery. *What is minimally invasive surgery?* 2001. Available from URL: http://www.mimis.com/whatis.html

37. Freud E, Zer M. Minimally invasive surgery in pediatric endocrinology *J Pediatr Endocrinol Metab* 2000; 13: 241–244.

38. Rao V, Freedom RM, Black MD. Minimally invasive surgery with cardioscopy for congenital heart defects. *Ann Thoracic Surg* 1999; 68: 1742–1745.

39. Rothenberg SS, Chang JH, Bealer JF. Experience with minimally invasive surgery in infants. *Am J Surg* 1998; 176: 654–658.

40. Waldhausen JH, Tapper D, Sawin RS. Minimally invasive surgery and clinical decision-making for pediatric malignancy. *Surg Endosc* 2000; 14: 250–253.

41. Yao D, Poppas DP. A clinical series of laparoscopic nephrectomy, nephroureterectomy and heminephroureterectomy in the pediatric population. *J Urol* 2000; 163: 1531–1535.

42. Firilas AM, Jackson RJ, Smith SD. Minimally invasive surgery: the pediatric surgery experience. *J Am Coll Surg* 1998; 186: 542–544.

43. Lugo-Vicente HL. Impact of minimally invasive surgery in children. *Bol Asoc Med PR* 1997; 89: 25–30.

44. Mahaffey SM, Davidoff AM, Oldham KT. Minimally invasive surgery: shortcut to recovery *Contemp Pediatr* 1994; 11: 102–104, 107–108.

45. Albanese CT, Harrison MR. Prenatal diagnosis and surgical intervention. In: Ashcraft KW, Murphy JP, Sharp RJ, Sigalet DL, Snyder CL. *Paediatric Surgery*, 3rd edn. Philadelphia: WB Saunders, 2000.

46. Weinzweig J, Panter KE, Pantaloni M, Spangenberger A, Harper JS, Lui F, James LF, Edstrom LE. The fetal cleft palate: 11. Scarless healing after *in utero* repair of a congenital model. *Plast Reconstr Surg* 1999; 104: 1356–1364.

47. Bruner JP, Tulipan NB, Richards WO, Walsh WF,

Boehm FH, Vrabcak EK. *In utero* repair of myelomeningocele: a comparison of endoscopy and hysterotomy. *Fetal Diagn Ther* 2000; 15: 83–88.

48. Tulipan N, Bruner JP, Hernanz-Schulman M, Lowe LH, Walsh WF, Nickolaus D, Oakes WJ. Effect of intrauterine myelomeningocele repair on central nervous system structure and function. *Pediatr Neurosurg* 1999; 31: 183–188.

49. Reddy VM, McElhinney DB. Update on prospects for fetal cardiovascular surgery. *Curr Opin Pediatr* 1997; 9: 530–535.

50. Quintero RA, Shukla AR, Homsy YL, Bukkapatnam R. Successful *in utero* endoscopic ablation of posterior urethral valves: a new dimension in fetal urology. *Urology Online* 2000; 55: 774.

51. Gonen R, Degani S, Kugelman A, Abend M, Bader D. Intrapartum drainage of fetal pleural effusion. *Prenat Diagn* 1999; 19: 1124–1126.

52. Kitano Y, Flake AW, Crombleholme TM, Johnson MP, Adzick NS. Open fetal surgery for life threatening fetal malformations. *Semin Perinatol* 1999; 23: 448–461.

53. Chiba T, Albanese CT, Jennings RW, Filly RA, Farrell JA, Harrison MR. *In utero* repair of rectal atresia after complete resection of a sacrococcygeal teratoma. *Fetal Diagn Ther* 2000; 15: 187–190.

54. Weinzweig J, Panter KE, Pantaloni M, Spangenberger A, Harper JS, Lui F, James LF, Edstrom LE. The fetal cleft palate: II. Scarless healing after *in utero* repair of a congenital model. *Plast Reconstr Surg* 1999; 104: 1356–1364.

55. Samuels P, Tan AK. Fetal scarless wound healing. *J Otolaryngol* 1999; 28: 296–302.

56. Vanhatalo S, van Nieuwenhuizen O. Fetal pain? *Brain Dev* 2000; 22: 145–150.

57. Montgomery WW. Surgery of the nasopharynx. In: Montgomery WW. *Surgery of the Upper Respiratory System*, 3rd edn. Baltimore: Williams & Wilkins, 1996.

58. Nieminen P, Tolonen U, Lopponen H. Snoring and obstructive sleep apnea in children: a 6-month follow-up study. *Arch Otolaryngol Head Neck Surg* 2000; 126: 481–486.

59. Suzuki M, Watanabe T, Mogi G. Clinical, bacteriological, and histological study of adenoids in children. *Am J Otolaryngol* 1999; 20: 85–90.

60. Davis CL, Chaliar A. Otolaryngological surgery. In: Phippen ML, Wells MP. *Patient Care During Operative and Invasive Procedures*. Philadelphia: WB Saunders, 2000.

61. Siddiqui N, Yung MW. Day-case adenoidectomy: how popular and safe in a rural environment? *J Laryngol Otol* 1997; 111: 444–446.

62. Chee NW, Chan KO. Clinical audit on tonsils and adenoid surgery. Is day surgery a reasonable option? *Ann Acad Med Singapore* 1996; 25: 245–242.

63. Holzmann D, Kaufmann T, Boesch M. On the

decision of outpatient adenoidectomy and adenotonsillectomy in children. *Int J Pediatr Otorhinolaryngol* 2000; 53: 9–16.

64. Vowles R, Loney E, Williams H, Gormley Fleming E, Kulkarni P, Ryan R. Is paediatric day case tonsillectomy desirable? The parents' perspective. *Int J Clin Pract* 2000; 54: 225–227.

65. Gabalski EC, Mattucci KF, Setzen M, Moleski P. Ambulatory tonsillectomy and adenoidectomy. *Laryngoscope* 1996; 106: 77–80.

66. Homer JJ, Williams BT, Semple P, Swanepoel A, Knight LC. Tonsillectomy by guillotine is less painful than by dissection. *Int J Pediatr Otorhinolaryngol* 2000; 52: 25–29.

67. Hultcrantz E, Linder A, Markstrom A. Tonsillectomy or tonsillotomy? A randomized study comparing postoperative pain and long-term effects. *Int J Pediatr Otorhinolaryngol* 1999; 51: 171–176.

68. Ochi K, Ohashi T, Sigiura N, Komatsuzaki Y, Okamoto A. Tonsillectomy using an ultrasonically activated scalpel. *Laryngoscope* 2000; 110: 1237–1238.

69. Robinson SR, Purdie GL. Reducing post-tonsillectomy pain with cryoanalgesia: a randomized controlled trial. *Laryngoscope* 2000; 110: 1128–1131.

70. Havas T. A longitudinal study of otitis media in the Aboriginal population of Groote Eylandt. *J Otolaryng Soc Austral* 1984; 5: 365–369.

71. Dugdale AE, Canty A, Lewis AN, Lovell S. The natural history of chronic middle ear disease in Australian Aboriginals: a cross-sectional study. *Med J Aust* 1978; 28 (suppl. March): 6–8.

72. Shields L. The influence of the family on young children's growth and disease at Cherbourg Aboriginal Community Australia. Thesis, University of Queensland, Brisbane, 1990.

73. Tonkin S. Maori infant health: 2. Study of morbidity and medico-social aspects. *NZ Med J* 1970; 72: 229–273.

74. Reed W, Struve S, Maynard JE. Otitis media and hearing deficiency among Eskimo children: a cohort study. *Am J Public Health* 967; 57: 1657–1662.

75. Johnson RL. Chronic otitis media in school age Navajo Indians. *Laryngoscope* 1967; 78: 1990–1995.

76. Serra AM. *Ear, Nose, and Throat Nursing*. Oxford: Blackwell, 1986.

77. Sigler BA, Schuring LT. *Ear, Nose and Throat Disorders*. St Louis: Mosby, 1993.

78. Wright KW, Spiegel PH. *Pediatric Ophthalmology and Strabismus*. St Louis: Mosby, 1999.

79. Mawhinney MS. Ophthalmic surgery. In: Meeker MH, Rothrock JC. *Alexander's Care of the Patient in Surgery*, 11th edn. Mosby: St Louis, 1999.

80. Abrahamsson M, Magnusson G, Sjostrand J. Inheritance of strabismus and the gain of using heredity to determine populations at risk of developing strabismus. *Acta Ophthalmol Scand* 1999; 77: 653–657.

81. Shields L. A comparative study of the care of hospitalized children in developed and developing countries. Thesis, University of Queensland, Brisbane,

1999. Available from URL: http://library.uq.edu.au/search/aShields+L/ashields+1/1,3,4,b/frameset&F=ashields+linda&1,,2

82. Decq P, Le Geurinel C, Palfi S, Djindjian M, Keravel Y, Nguyen JP. A new device for endoscopic third ventriculostomy. *J Neurosurg* 2000; 93: 509–512.

83. Cordier PL, Sion B. Positioning the patient. In: Phippen ML, Wells MP. *Patient Care during Operative and Invasive Procedures*. Philadelphia: WB Saunders, 2000.

84. Kerner M. Neurosurgery. In: Phippen ML, Wells MP. *Patient Care During Operative and Invasive Procedures*. Philadelphia: WB Saunders 2000.

85. Gruber DP, Brockmeyer DL, Walker ML. Head injuries in children. In: Ashcraft KW, Murphy JP, Sharp RJ, Sigalet DL, Snyder CL. *Pediatric Surgery*, 3rd edn. Philadelphia: WB Saunders, 2000.

86. Morris JK, Wald NJ. Quantifying the decline in the birth prevalence of neural tube defects in England and Wales. *J Med Screen* 1999; 6: 182–185.

87. Molloy AM, Mills JL, Kirke PN, Weir DG, Scott JM. Folate status and neural tube defects in England and Wales. *J Med Screen* 1991; 6: 182–185.

88. Petsonk EL. Couriers of asthma: antigenic proteins in natural rubber latex. *Occup Med* 2000; 15: 421–430.

89. Murphy M, Hahn GV. Orthopedic surgery. In: Phippen ML, Wells MP. *Patient Care during Operative and Invasive Procedures*. Philadelphia: WB Saunders, 2000.

90. Williams PF, Cole WG. *Orthopaedic Management in Childhood*. London: Chapman & Hall, 1991.

91. Arndt CAS. Neoplasms of bone. In: Behrman RE, Kliegman RM, Jenson HB eds. *Nelson Textbook of Paediatrics*, 16th edn. Philadelphia: WB Saunders 2000.

92. Thompson GH, Scoles PV. Bone and joint disorders. In: Behrman RE, Kliegman RM, Jenson HB eds. *Nelson Textbook of Pediatrics*, 16th edn. Philadelphia: WB Saunders, 2000.

93. Golden A, Low DW. Plastic surgery. In: Phippen ML, Wells MP. *Patient Care during Operative and Invasive Procedures*. Philadelphia: WB Saunders, 2000.

94. David DJ, Simpson DA. Craniosynostosis. In: Mustard, JC, Jackson IT eds. *Plastic Surgery in Infancy and Childhood*, 3rd edn. Edinburgh: Churchill Livingstone, 1988.

95. Colohan ART, Persing, IA, Edgerton J, Edgerton MT. Encephalocele. In: Mustard, JC, Jackson IT eds. *Plastic Surgery in Infancy and Childhood*, 3rd edn. Edinburgh: Churchill Livingstone, 1988.

96. Johnsen D, Tinanoff N. The oral cavity: cleft lip and palate. In: Behrman RE, Kliegman RM, Jenson HB eds. *Nelson Textbook of Pediatrics*, 16th edn. Philadelphia: WB Saunders, 2000.

97. Bender PL. Genetics of cleft lip and palate. *J Pediatr Nurs* 2000; 15: 242–249.

98. Jackson IT. Cleft lip and palate. In: Mustard, JC, Jackson IT eds. *Plastic Surgery in Infancy and Childhood*, 3rd edn. Edinburgh: Churchill Livingstone, 1988.

99. Palmer B. Correction of prominent ears. In: Mustard,

JC, Jackson IT eds. *Plastic Surgery in Infancy and Childhood*, 3rd edn. Edinburgh: Churchill Livingstone, 1988.

100. Caouette-Laberge L, Guay N, Bortoluzzi P, Belleville C. Otoplasty: anterior scoring technique acid results in 500 cases. *Plast Reconstr Surg* 2000; 105: 504–515.

101. Bartley J. How long should ears be bandaged after otoplasty? *J Laryngol Otol* 1998; 112: 531–532.

102. Lister GD. Upper extremity. In: Mustard, JC, Jackson IT eds. *Plastic Surgery in Infancy and Childhood*, 3rd edn. Edinburgh: Churchill Livingstone, 1988.

103. Laberge JM, Nguyen LT, Shaw KS. Teratomas, dermoids and other soft tissue tumours. In: Ashcraft KW, Murphy JP, Sharp RJ, Sigalet DL, Snyder CL. *Paediatric Surgery*, 3rd edn. Philadelphia: MT Saunders, 2000.

104. Jaksic T, Nigro JF, Hicks MJ. Nevus and melanoma. In: Ashcraft KW, Murphy JP, Sharp RJ, Sigalet DL, Snyder CL. *Paediatric Surgery*, 3rd edn. Philadelphia: MT Saunders, 2000.

105. Stringel G. Hemangiomas and lymphangiomas. In: Ashcraft KW, Murphy JP, Sharp RJ, Sigalet DL, Snyder CL. *Paediatric Surgery*, 3rd edn. Philadelphia: MT Saunders, 2000.

106. Shan E, Bahar-Fuchs SA, Abu-Hammad I, Friger M, Rosenberg L. A burn prevention program as a long-term investment: trends in burn injuries among Jews and Bedouin children in Israel. *Burns* 2000; 26: 171–177.

107. El-Badawy A, Mabrouk AR. Epidemiology of childhood burns in the burn unit of Ain Shams University in Cairo, Egypt. *Burns* 1998; 24: 728–732.

108. Elisdottir R, Ludvigsson P, Einarsson O, Thorgrimsson S, Haraldsson A. Paediatric burns in Iceland. Hospital admissions 1982–1995, a populations based study. *Burns* 1999; 25: 149–151.

109. Cerovac S, Roberts AH. Burns sustained by hot bath and shower water. *Burns* 2000; 26: 251–259.

110. Kidsafe Australia. *Facts sheet: scalds safety*. Available from URL: http://www.kidsafe.com.au/scalds.pdf

111. Smith T. Accidents, poisoning and violence as a cause of hospital admissions in children. *Health Bull Edinb* 1991; 49: 237–244.

112. Mott SR, Fazekas NF, James SR. *Nursing Care of Children and Families*. Menlo Park: Addison Wesley, 1985.

113. Sharp RJ. Burns. In: Ashcraft KW, Murphy JP, Sharp RJ, Sigalet DL, Snyder CL. *Paediatric Surgery*, 3rd edn. Philadelphia: MT Saunders, 2000.

114. Grous C, Cendron M. Urological surgery. In: Phippen ML, Wells MP. *Patient Care during Operative and Invasive Procedures*. Philadelphia: WB Saunders, 2000.

115. Hendren WH. Urethral valves. In: Ashcraft KW, Murphy JP, Sharp RJ, Sigalet DL, Snyder CL. *Paediatric Surgery*, 3rd edn. Philadelphia: MT Saunders, 2000.

116. Coplen DE, Snyder HM. Ureteral obstruction and malformations. In: Ashcraft KW, Murphy JP, Sharp RJ, Sigalet DL, Snyder CL. *Paediatric Surgery*, 3rd edn. Philadelphia: MT Saunders, 2000.

117. Motoyama EK, Davis PJ. *Smith's Anaesthesia for Infants and Children*, 6th edn. St Louis: Mosby, 1996.

118. Hughes DG. Monitoring in paediatric anaesthesia. In: Mather SJ, Hughes DG eds. *A Hand Book of Paediatric Anaesthesia*, 2nd edn. Oxford: Oxford University Press, 1996.

119. MIMS Pharmaceutical database. *EMLA*. Available from URL: http://intranet.mater.org.au/mims/DSPPROD.ASP?ACT=DSPC&MRN=1901&KEY=95

120. Hughes DG. Pain management in children. In: Mather SJ, Hughes DG eds. *A Hand Book of Paediatric Anaesthesia*, 2nd edn. Oxford: Oxford University Press, 1996.

121. Morgan GE, Mikhail MS. *Clinical Anesthesiology*, 2nd edn. Stamford: Appleton & Lange, 1996.

122. *Competency Standards for Perioperative Nurses*. Sydney: Australian Confederation of Operating Room Nurses, 1999.

123. Meyer-Pahoulis E. Pediatric postanesthesia care. *Plastic Surgical Nursing* 1994; 14: 92–95.

Surgical procedures on children

Perioperative midwifery | 5

11 | Procedures conducted within the obstetric operating theatre environment

Amanda Silvey

OVERVIEW

The labour process and childbirth experience is often referred to as a normal and natural life event for women. While this is true for most women, it is important to note that the experience is always unique for all women and can be extremely variable from one pregnancy to the next. Progress in labour is not always predictable and unanticipated responses, either maternal or fetal, can occur at any time. Given this, a seemingly normal labour can quickly change course, becoming complicated and, in some cases, necessitate emergency intervention. This may include delivery by emergency Caesarean section (C/S), by forceps or by Ventouse extraction (where appropriate) to ensure a safe and positive outcome for both mother and baby. For this reason alone, most tertiary-level birthing facilities and delivery units have an operating room (OR) available on site, or at least in close proximity. The obstetric OR can be utilised for both elective and acute operative or invasive procedures. Some of these include C/S and instrumental deliveries, which encompass methods using forceps or Ventouse extraction.

OBSTETRIC OPERATIVE PROCEDURES

Table 11.1 shows some of the more commonly performed obstetric operative procedures. In some situations, instrumental deliveries will be attempted in the OR environment, particularly if the condition of the mother or baby is such that urgent delivery is required should these methods fail. If there is a high possibility that delivery may have to be by C/S, the terms 'trial of forceps delivery' or a 'trial of Ventouse extraction' apply. The woman, her support person and all staff involved are prepared accordingly and will be ready to proceed to C/S immediately if required. This means scrub personnel are set up and waiting. The anaesthetic team is organised, as is the obstetric and midwifery team. A paediatrician is usually required at all emergency deliveries where known fetal or maternal conditions or abnormalities complicate a pregnancy.

TUBAL LIGATION

Although this procedure is normally performed as a gynaecological procedure, it can be done as an additional procedure at the time of elective C/S if the necessary legal and ethical arrangements have been made in advance. While tubal ligation is a reversible procedure, it is important to note that consent and organisation for this procedure will only be made following extensive counselling of the woman and her partner (if applicable). Previously, many women requesting the procedure underwent postpartum sterilisation via minilaparotomy, which took place approximately 24 hours post delivery. This fell into disfavour because of the requirement for postpartum general anaesthesia (GA). This in turn posed some restrictions on mobilisation after an otherwise normal delivery, thereby increasing the risk of pulmonary embolism. In addition, sterilisation at the

> **Table 11.1**
> **Common obstetric operative procedures**
>
> - **Forceps delivery**: involves the application of one of three types of forceps to the fetal head. The type chosen depends on the position of the fetus in the pelvis, the surrounding clinical findings and labour progress
> - **Ventouse extraction**: a suction cup is applied to the fetal head and, as for forceps delivery, traction is then used to deliver the baby vaginally. It is not always necessary to conduct such deliveries in the OR
> - **Episiotomy**: while not always necessary, an episiotomy is sometimes performed before delivery by forceps or Ventouse delivery
> - **Emergency hysterectomy**: performed only as a last resort in emergencies where maternal bleeding cannot be controlled by other measures and the mother's life is therefore at risk. It can follow either a C/S or vaginal delivery
> - **Evacuation of a vulval or perineal haematoma**: An incision is made to release the collection of blood/haematoma. A drain may be placed temporarily to prevent recollection
> - **Surgical repair of the perineum:** following a traumatic vaginal delivery of where a third-degree tear of episiotomy has resulted
> - **Examination under anaesthetic (EUA)**: an EUA may be indicated to investigate *post-partum* bleeding or in cases or a retained placenta, placental tissue or membranes. This involves a manual examination *per vaginam* of the uterine wall, cervix and uterus, and usually will be performed under a general anaesthetic
> - **Emergency laparotomy**: to investigate postoperative bleeding or postdelivery bleeding/wound dehiscence or possible uterine rupture
> - **Insertion or extraction of cervical sutures**: insertion of a 'cervical stitch' is offered to women with a history of late miscarriage in a previous pregnancy or for women with known cases of cervical incompetence. The stitch is removed later in pregnancy, usually in the third trimester unless indicated before this time. Because the stitch is quite thick in diameter, it is more like a tape in appearance

time of delivery is more likely associated with future regret. Ideally, consent should be obtained well before delivery at some point during the antenatal period as it is unlikely that a woman can give informed consent if making this decision or request when in labour.

EXTERNAL CEPHALIC VERSION

This occurs where the fetus is manually rotated by the obstetrician during abdominal palpation to change the position of the baby from breech to a cephalic presentation. Before this is attempted, the amniotic fluid sac must be intact and there must be plenty of amniotic fluid surrounding the baby – an ultrasound can confirm this. Artificial rupture of membranes (ARM) will often be performed immediately following this and an intravenous (IV) Syntocinon infusion commenced to establish regular uterine contractions to augment labour and help maintain the fetal position. The aim of performing an ARM following a successful external cephalic version is to maintain the baby in the cephalic presentation.

ABNORMAL DELIVERY

Abnormal delivery includes any of the following.

- Instrumental delivery.
- Ventouse extraction.
- C/S.

Instrumental and Ventouse delivery are not necessarily performed within the OR. The decision to perform the above delivery methods in an operative environment lies with the obstetric team and is dependent on labour history, progress, and maternal and fetal status to date. To attempt delivery in case of forceps or Ventouse extraction, a number of criteria must be met. It is essential that the cervix has reached full dilatation of 10 cm and is fully effaced (thinned out). This criterion does not apply to C/S. Instrumental delivery and Ventouse extraction are implemented to expedite delivery.

Some of the more common indications for intervention include the following.[1]

- Fetal distress.
- Lack of progression in the first or second stage of labour.
- Malposition of the fetus.

- Maternal conditions such as pre-eclampsia, cardiac and neurological conditions, or respiratory conditions where excessive maternal effort needs to be avoided.

ANAESTHETICS IN OBSTETRICS

Owing to the physiological and physical changes that occur in pregnancy, the risk of anaesthetic-related complications increases significantly. Where possible, operative procedures on pregnant women are performed under an epidural block or spinal block, or a combination of the two. Only in extreme emergencies, specific maternal request or following a failed spinal or epidural anaesthetic is a general anaesthetic considered by the anaesthetist.

CAESAREAN SECTION (C/S)

C/S is the surgical technique whereby the fetus is delivered through an incision in the uterus.[2] C/S is becoming a controversial issue in obstetrics.[3] There has been a steady rise in the incidence of C/S in most developing countries over the past 20–30 years.[4] Interestingly, the rate of performance of this procedure is significantly higher in the private sector. Indicators and influencing factors for this mode of delivery are considerable.[5,6] Although maternal haemorrhage is still considered the most probable causative factor in the majority of maternal deaths,[2] improved skills in the area of both general and regional anaesthesia has made C/S a safer event.

In addition, expectant parents are now taking more of an active approach in preparing for pregnancy and the childbirth experience. Increased attendance and awareness through antenatal education has prompted a desire to participate in decision-making with regard to their own obstetric management and care. It can be suggested that increasing numbers of women are opting for repeat C/S in subsequent pregnancies rather than attempting a trial vaginal delivery.[7]

Depending on the circumstances, most women can go on to have a successful vaginal delivery following a previous C/S birth. The main risk factor, however, is the possibility of uterine rupture during labour, although the incidence is low.[8]

Fear of litigation on the part of medical and other health professionals can be a contributing factor to decisions about the appropriateness of C/S.[2] Media focus toward moral issues surrounding both maternal rights and the rights of the unborn fetus add further pressure. All of these contribute to the escalating occurrence of this procedure. While the rate is variable depending greatly on country, population, facilities and labour management style, in most tertiary teaching maternity centres the incidence of C/S is now almost 15–25%.[2] This demonstrates a dramatic increase compared with figures recorded two decades ago, when C/S occurred at approximately 5–10% of all recorded births,[2] though in some countries the rate of C/S is declining.[9]

INDICATIONS FOR C/S

Table 11.2 shows the indications for C/S.

COMPLICATIONS AND RISKS FROM DELIVERY BY C/S

- **Maternal**: the risks that apply to all major surgery further increase the maternal mortality rate when compared with that of spontaneous vaginal delivery.
- Other considerations are the expected increased blood loss – normal estimated blood loss for C/S is about 600 ml as opposed to an expected blood loss of up to 400 ml at vaginal birth.
- Risk of infection secondary to surgical intervention.

The most frequent associated complications to consider are the following.

- **Haemorrhage**: 6% of maternal deaths are associated with C/S.[10] The risks increase in pregnancies complicated with conditions such as placenta praevia, placental abruption, prolonged labour, polyhydramnios and grand multiparity.
- **Bladder injury**: the risk of bladder injury during C/S is relatively low but is higher in an emergency C/S (especially if labour was prolonged) and in repeat C/S where the bladder can sometimes be adherent to the lower uterine segment. Here, bladder injury may be sustained during attempts to divide or dissect adhesions or scarring.[11] The introduction of an indwelling catheter preoperatively to maintain an empty bladder will assist in reducing injury or trauma, while also

Table 11.2
Indications for Caesarean section[2]

- Previous Caesarean section is most common indicator – 40%
- Dystocia – obstructed labour/contracted pelvis – 20%
- Fetal distress – 12%
- Breech presentation – 10%
- Other malpresentations:
  - oblique or transverse lie
  - brow or face
  - compound
- Cord prolapse
- Antepartum haemorrhage
- Placental abruption
- Placenta praevia
- Pre-eclampsia
- Evidence of uterine rupture
- Severe intrauterine growth retardation
- Severe oligohydramnios
- Multiple pregnancies
- Cephalopelvic disproportion: macrosomic infant
- Hydrocephaly
- Rhesus isoimmunisation:
  - medical indications:
    - neurological/cardiac or renal disease processes
    - tumour
    - active genital herpes
  - elective – with or without indication: delivery of an infant following an intrauterine fetal death/maternal request

providing more space for delivery of the baby. The assistant can also aid in reducing bladder trauma by providing adequate exposure to the lower uterine segment through correct placement of a retractor such as the Balfour Doyen or similar.

- **Wound infection**: as with all major surgery, the potential for postoperative wound infection after a C/S is a reality. The use of prophylactic antibiotics has been shown to decrease the risk of postoperative febrile morbidity.[10] These are given as a single IV dose by the anaesthetist intraoperatively following delivery of the baby.
- While variables will influence the rate, on average a wound infection will occur in approximately 1–9% of cases.[10] The incidence is likely to increase with premature rupture of membranes (PROM) and/or when prolonged labour has occurred or where maternal anaemia existed preoperatively. Usually, the infection is with common pathogens, often a mixture of anaerobic and aerobic bacteria.

Implementation and adherence to infection control measures will minimise the risk of infection. Some of these measures include:
- preoperative skin preparation;
- removal of abdominal and suprapubic hair using clippers rather than a shaver;
- utilisation of disposable drapes in preference to linen drapes if possible;
- strict adherence to observation of aseptic techniques;
- limiting movement within the OR environment; and
- restricting the number of staff and support people in the OR to a minimum.
- **Chest infections** can be a complication following major surgery, even in healthy young women. When smoking, obesity or respiratory tract infections are present or a general anaesthetic performed, chest infections may occur more frequently.

- **Endometritis**: poses a much higher threat following C/S when compared with a normal vaginal delivery (NVD).[9]
- **Urinary tract infections**: can result following any invasive renal or bladder procedure. At C/S, the preoperative placement of an indwelling urinary catheter is routine. Following closure post-C/S, some practitioners will introduce a 'swab' per vaginum to evacuate any clots after first massaging the uterus. These are potential sources of infection into the genitourinary tract.
- **Thromboembolism** is responsible for a significant percentage of maternal deaths that occur after C/S. The risk of developing deep vein thrombosis (DVT) is almost five times higher than that of development after a NVD.[12]

NEONATAL RISKS

Babies born by C/S are at greater risk of respiratory distress syndrome, secondary to the retention of fetal lung fluid. In an NVD, this fluid is expelled during compression of the thoracic cavity in the birth process. In C/S, this does not occur. As soon as the infant's head is delivered, adequate suctioning of the mouth and oropharynx is essential to reduce the risk of inhalation of fluids into the lungs. (The scrub nurse is usually responsible for this.)

PREPARING THE WOMAN FOR C/S

When a booking is made for an elective C/S, the accuracy of the estimated date of confinement is important. In terms of gestation, 1–2 weeks can have a considerable impact on the management decisions and affect outcome for the baby. Should early delivery occur and the mother's dates are uncertain, comparison of data from clinical observations is considered to assist in establishing approximate gestation.

- Ultrasound.
- Fundal height.
- Fetal growth.

Bookings for elective C/Ss are usually scheduled between 38 and 39 weeks of pregnancy. Should the woman spontaneously labour or rupture her membranes before this date, the procedure will be performed as an emergency.

For planned elective cases

The woman will be admitted the evening before or on the day of surgery. In either case, the woman will have fasted overnight – no food or fluids for at least 6 hours. Bowel preparation is no longer routine, but its use will depend on the hospital facility in question. On arrival, a history is obtained and abdominal palpation performed to confirm cephalic or breech presentation. This is particularly important in primigravid women to determine the need for C/S. If the indication for C/S was for breech presentation a baseline set of observations – vital signs including blood pressure, pulse rate, respiratory rate and temperature – are recorded and the fetal heart rate (FHR) auscultated. Appropriate blood tests are done including a full blood count (FBC) and cross-matching (unless otherwise indicated), and routine urine tests are also performed at this point.

The woman will be asked to don appropriate operative attire following a preoperative shower. In some hospitals, a suprapubic shave (using clippers or similar) is performed-as close to surgery as possible. The insertion of an indwelling catheter is also required before surgery, but is often attended to following anaesthetic preparation.

ANAESTHESIA FOR C/S AND OTHER OBSTETRIC PROCEDURES

Obstetric anaesthesia is a specialised area of practice. As mentioned above, GA is avoided where possible in pregnancy. The majority of procedures including C/S are performed under epidural or spinal block. The application of a combined spinal–epidural has become more popular in recent years and the operative procedure is performed under a spinal anaesthetic, however, an epidural catheter is placed at the same time as the spinal block insertion and can be accessed accordingly should the spinal block fail to provide adequate anaesthesia. Where spinal anaesthesia fails and in the absence of epidural catheter placement, a GA is the only option. An added benefit of the combined spinal–epidural is the ability to provide additional pain relief should it be necessary in the postoperative period. The option for a bolus epidural top up or postoperative infusion is available. Post-C/S, the epidural catheter is usually left in

Procedures conducted within the obstetric operating theatre environment

place until just before transfer from the recovery room to the postnatal ward.

PREOPERATIVELY

As part of the anaesthetic preparation, the woman will have been prescribed an H_2-antagonist such as Ranitidine to decrease the production of acid and to increase the pH of the stomach contents. In emergencies, the woman will be given sodium citrate or similar before surgery to neutralise gastric acids. Additionally, an antiemetic such as metaclopramide may be administered to speed up gastric emptying. This decreases the risk of Mendelson's acid aspiration syndrome, to which pregnant women are more prone due to the displacement of the stomach and other abdominal organs as a result of the gravid uterus.[2]

It is worth noting that if IV access is required in the obstetric patient for any reason, nothing less than a 16g catheter is used. If haemorrhage does occur, IV access is vital and fluids need to be replaced rapidly as a life-saving measure. For elective and emergency C/S, an IV line will be established in the first instance. One litre of normal saline or a similar solution (such as Hartmann's) will be infused before either spinal or epidural placement to counteract the anticipated fall in blood pressure that may result.[9]

In most centres the anaesthetist will be assisted by an anaesthetic technician or a nurse or midwife for the duration of the anaesthetic. Monitoring equipment will have been applied to the woman following insertion of the IV line.

Epidural catheter placement/spinal block

This procedure can be done in either a sitting or lying position (usually on the operating table) depending on the anaesthetist's preference. This is not an easy procedure to perform in pregnant women, so careful positioning is essential. Maintaining an appropriate position can be challenging for the woman if she is already in labour and is having to contend with contractions during the procedure.

Because of this, good communication between the anaesthetist and the woman is important. The anaesthetist will explain everything he/she is about to do and the woman is asked to alert staff to impending contractions as they occur. The midwife or support person can provide much needed support by helping maintain the position as well as comfort and distraction at this time. Once the desired level of epidural or spinal block has been achieved, with the anaesthetist's permission, the woman is appropriately positioned on the operating table. When lying in a supine position in later pregnancy (usually after 34 weeks), the weight of the pregnant uterus can cause aortocaval compression. The resulting effects can compromise both the mother and foetus. To prevent this from occurring, the woman is positioned accordingly. Either the operating table itself is tilted laterally or a foam wedge is placed usually under the woman's right hip. This position is maintained right through the operation until delivery of the baby.

Once the anaesthetist is satisfied that an appropriate block has been achieved and vital signs are stable, an indwelling catheter can be inserted, sometimes beforehand. With the surgical team prepared and waiting, the woman can be transferred into the OR.

Other procedures

If the woman is already in labour, the FHR will be auscultated intermittently or a continuous carditocograph (fetal monitor) will be in progress. This monitor demonstrates the FHR and uterine activity and provides a good indicator of fetal status during the antenatal period and/or in labour.

SUPPORT PERSONS

The value of this role is often underestimated. An important aspect of the development of a positive birthing experience for the mother is that of the emotional and sometimes physical support received throughout her labour and delivery. While the expectant father (the woman's husband or partner) usually fulfils this supportive role, it would be wise to use caution when acknowledging or addressing the support person at delivery. Depending on the social and family dynamics, the person/persons in this role could vary from partners to relatives, from ex-partners to new partners, to older children, close friends or a combination of all. Whatever the situation, the support people are there to offer much needed encouragement, inspiration, reassurance, comfort and coaching to the woman at one of the most vulnerable moments of her life. It can be a rewarding experience for all participants invited to share in such a special event.

Role of the support person at C/S

Except in cases of extreme emergency or where GA is anticipated at C/S, it is usual for the support person(s) (usually limited to one person) to accompany the woman into the OR and remain with her for the duration of the procedure. For the support person, walking into such an unfamiliar environment can be a rather daunting experience. If time permits, providing a brief orientation to the actual OR and equipment is beneficial and more likely to reduce some of this anxiety. It may help if the support people are made aware of what is going to happen ahead of time, and an explanation regarding staff roles and the sequence of events is offered. Knowing that certain practices are routine, such as taking the baby immediately to the resuscitaire following delivery, also helps.

The following lists other useful information to offer the partner or support person.

- Length of the operation.
- Where you can move within the theatre.
- Theatre attire: correct wearing of face masks and hats, etc.
- What to do if feeling faint at any time and where to go.
- What to expect after the operation: transfer to the recovery room and length of stay.
- What happens to the baby.

It is important to remind the support person and family members that even though the procedure is being conducted while the woman is awake, she is actually undergoing major abdominal surgery and will have postoperative and recovery needs just as general postoperative patients do, and in the weeks following surgery she will also have the needs of her new baby to attend to.

Staff involved in C/S

- Anaesthetic team of two or three: consultant/registrar/anaesthetics technician.
- Circulating midwife.
- Scrub nurse/midwife.
- Surgeon and assistant.
- Paediatrician: depends on the facility but may <u>not</u> always be required at elective C/S:
  - where presentation is normal; or
  - + or – neonatal nursing staff.

Staff numbers increase depending on need, particularly in cases of multiple pregnancy.

Procedure

Once the woman is in the OR, the operative site is prepared using a skin preparation and her abdomen square-draped. The surgeon will usually prefer to participate in this as he/she needs to identify some anatomical landmarks such as iliac crests before they are hidden by drapes. This is done so that a symmetrical and aesthetically suitable skin incision can be done. A thyroid screen or similar is raised and kept high enough to maintain the sterile field and keep the drapes off the woman's face, but low enough to allow the support person to watch the delivery should they so choose. The scrub nurse/midwife positions the Mayo table and instrument trolley at the foot of the bed and usually stands opposite the surgeon on the woman's left side. The assistant stands next to the scrub nurse. Suction (double suction is useful) will be positioned at either the foot of the operating table or the side.

Instruments required for C/S

These instruments are similar to those required for major abdominal surgery, with additional instruments specific to obstetrics and gynaecology. Most facilities will have a specific instrument set they use for C/S and although these will vary from place to place, the instruments in Figures 11.1–11.4 and Tables 11.3–11.8 are considered essential.

Diathermy is not usually required for C/S but may be used according to the surgeon's preference. However, it must be available for unanticipated haemorrhage and is always used for cases of known

Procedures conducted within the obstetric operating theatre environment

Table 11.3
Example of a standard Caesarean section tray

- **No. 4 scalpel handles** × 2
- **Fine medium and heavy-toothed dissection forceps** × 3 (these may include Gilles, Lanes or Bonney's forceps)
- **Long plain packing forceps** × 1
- **Fine plain forceps** (such as Waugh's)
- **Plain dressing forceps** × 1
- **Heavy Mayo scissors curved** × 2
- **Heavy Mayo scissors straight** × 1 (or similar, to use in cutting the umbilical cord)
- **Fine curved scissors** (such as McIndoe, for use on finer tissues, for example at tubal ligation)
- **Suture scissors straight** × 1
- **Suture scissors curved** × 1
- **Kocher forceps curved** × 2 (used mainly to clamp, sometimes double clamp, the umbilical cord at delivery and to assist in the gentle guiding out of placental membranes which can sometimes be slightly adherent to the uterine wall)
- **Kocher forceps straight** × 2
- **Green–Armytage forceps** × 6 (applied on the mouth of the uterus after delivery of the baby and placenta, aiding in control of blood loss and in identifying anatomically the uterine edges before repair/closure of the uterus)
- **Criles–Armytage forceps** × 10
- **Rampley sponge holding forceps** × 3 (used as skin preparation and to hold small swabs)
- **Medium to large curved retractor** × 1 (such as Doyen or similar and positioned under the symphysis pubis to provide exposure to the bladder and lower uterine segment before uterine incision and used for general retraction throughout the procedure)
- **Small to medium retractor** × 1
- **Backhaus towel clips** × 6
- **Mayo needle holders** × 3
- **Wrigley's obstetric forceps** × 1 pair
- **Yankuer sucker or Poole sucker**

Note that the use of metal suckers will vary from place to place, but in general, use of the suction tubing alone for the suction of amniotic fluid and blood is the norm. Poole suckers should be available in the theatre though and opened as required.

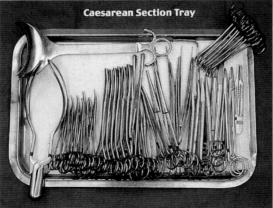

Fig. 11.1 Instruments used for C/S

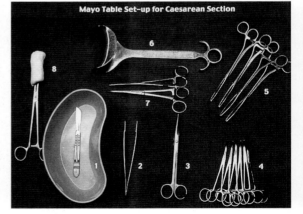

Fig. 11.2 Mayo table set-up for C/S

Table 11.4
Example of a Mayo table map

- Sharps container with scalpel handle with 22 blade attached × 1
- Heavy-toothed forceps × 1
- Heavy-curved dissecting scissors × 1
- Suture scissors × 1
- Criles artery forceps × 6
- Large Doyen retractor or similar × 1
- Green–Armytage forceps × 6
- Rampley sponge holder with small gauze swab attached (referred to as a 'swab on a stick')

Table 11.5
Extra items on the instrument trolley

- One pair of Wrigley's obstetric forceps
- Extra 'swabs on sticks'
- Loaded sutures for the repairing/closing of the uterus
- Instruments and suction catheter for the baby (this includes: Kocher forceps × 2, scissors for cutting the umbilical cord and a disposable cord clamp)

Table 11.6
Other equipment required by the scrub nurse/midwife

Bowl sets should include:

- Splash bowls × 2 (one for the surgeon)
- Large bowl for containing soiled swabs
- Sharps container
- Small bowls
- Large kidney dishes × 3 (can be used to contain instruments for cutting cord clamp and receiving placenta, wet and dry sponges)

Table 11.7
Standard extras required

- Warm sterile water for splash bowls (2 litres)
- No 22 blades
- Large abdominal sponges × 10
- Small gauze swabs × 5
- Disposable suction tubing
- Infant suction catheter (size 10 fg for term infant, 8 fg for the premature infant)
- T-connector or similar (to attach the infant suction catheter to the suction tubing)
- Disposable cord clamp
- Suture material as per the surgeon's preference
- Suture mat
- Dressing material as per the surgeon's preference

Procedures conducted within the obstetric operating theatre environment

Procedures conducted within the obstetric operating theatre environment

Table 11.8 **Extras to have at hand**

- Additional large sponges and small swabs
- Catgut ties
- Extra suction tubing/suction equipment
- Poole suction
- Hysterectomy tray
- Redivac drain or similar

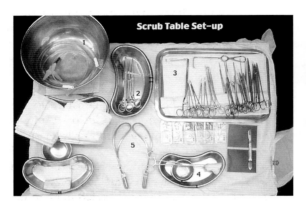

Fig. 11.3 Scrub table set-up

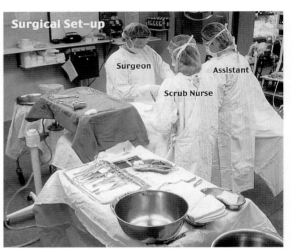

Fig. 11.4 Surgical set-up

placenta praevia, uterine rupture and placental abruption.

In such cases it is important to have Carboprost (**Prostin/15m**) available, a refrigerated drug sometimes used to control severe bleeding of the uterus, in the OR. It can be injected directly into the myometrium or intramuscularly.

Length of procedure

C/S takes on average 30–45 minutes from start to finish although this will depend on the speed and skill of the surgeon. The baby is usually delivered within the first few minutes of surgery.

Operation

Abdominal wall incision

The Pfannenstiel incision is used in most cases for C/S.

Advantages

- Cosmetic: the scar is low and can be hidden by pubic hair and bikini pant.

- Lower risk of wound dehiscence and incisional hernia.
- Less postoperative pain.

Disadvantages

- Takes a little longer particularly at repeat C/S as scarring may delay separation of the rectus sheath from the rectus abdominal muscles, which then require separation before incision into the peritoneum vertically.
- Not suitable for complicated cases such as laparotomy to explore haemorrhage.

Vertical subumbilical incision

The vertical subumbilical incision is used more if the need for emergency delivery is extreme such as cord prolapse or severe fetal distress or in cases where hysterectomy or a classical C/S is indicated such as a grade 4 placental praevia.

Advantages

- Provides better exposure and vision for the surgeon.
- Associated with less blood loss.

Transverse uterine incision

This is the most common technique – > 90% where a transverse incision is made throughout the lower segment of the uterus after opening the peritoneal cavity.[2] The incidence of wound dehiscence following this method is extremely small – as low as 1%.[10]

Vertical lower uterine incision

A vertical midline incision is made into the lower uterine segment. It is infrequently used but like a 'classical C/S' may be chosen in cases where a transverse incision is not possible, e.g. in a poorly formed lower uterine segment or in the presence of a contraction ring, which unless cut, inhibits delivery of the baby. In this incision type, there is the risk of inadvertently extending the incision downward. If this occurs, tears through the cervix and into the vagina are possibilities as is trauma to the bladder.[12]

Upper segment C/S

Classical C/S

A vertical midline incision is made into the muscle of the upper uterine segment. This is rarely used but can be the required method in a small percentage of cases.

- Transverse lie of the fetus.
- Delivery of an infant of extremely immature gestation where no or little formation of the lower uterine segment is apparent.
- In some cases of placenta praevia or where large vessels are present over the lower segment.

In this method, wound closure is more difficult and therefore repair takes longer. The development of adhesions seems to be greater as is the incidence of infection. Overall risk of rupture after a classical C/S increases to approximately 6% compared with that for a lower segment transverse incision.

Classical C/S is also associated with poorer wound healing and wound dehiscence.[2,10,12]

OPERATION PROCEDURE FOR LOWER UTERINE SEGMENT C/S

Transverse incision

- Skin is incised using a **Pfannenstiel incision**.
- Subcutaneous fat is divided with blunt scissors or the fingers.
- Rectus sheath is incised: the abdominal rectus muscle is dissected from the rectus sheath to enable an approach into the abdominal cavity.
- Peritoneum is divided with dissecting scissors. Sometimes the peritoneum is elevated using two artery forceps: if this is done, the surgeon must ensure that the bowel or omentum is not inadvertently included.
- Small incision with sharp scissors opens the parietal peritoneum. At this point, moist packs are sometimes positioned on either side of the uterus to limit blood and amniotic fluid loss from entering the peritoneal cavity.
- Lower uterine segment is now exposed. It is worth noting that due to physiological displacement, the uterus is sometimes slightly rotated more to the right side. With this in mind, the surgeon is in a better position to avoid angle tears when making the incision into the lower segment.
- Doyen retractor (or similar) is positioned under the symphysis pubis to expose the lower segment and the bladder.
- Visceral peritoneum is dissected sharply about 2–3 cm above the bladder. In a repeat C/S, it may take longer to release adhesions from previous scarring.
- Using the fingers, the surgeon reflects the bladder off the lower uterine segment to avoid bladder trauma or damage to congested venous plexuses.
- A 10–12-cm incision is then made into the lower uterine segment, with a slight upward curve at each end. This is done to reduce the risk of angle tears, which could extend to and involve the uterine arteries.
- Amniotic fluid and blood are released and suctioned accordingly.
- At this point, the baby can be delivered.
- In a cephalic presentation, the surgeon will deliver the baby by placing a hand into the uterine cavity, supporting the presenting part. The assistant helps in delivery of the baby by applying extra abdominal pressure to the uterine fundus.

Procedures conducted within the obstetric operating theatre environment

- On delivery of the head, the oropharynx is suctioned of amniotic fluid/blood/mucus or meconium to reduce the risk of inhalation aspiration of any of these into the lungs. This is normally attended to by the scrub/midwife.
- When the rest of the baby has been born, the scrub nurse/midwife offers equipment to clamp and cut the cord. A disposable cord clamp is applied (approximately 1.5–2.0 cm from umbilical cord base), a second clamp, usually a Kocher forceps (or similar), is placed and the cord cut. The baby will then be received into warm sterile wraps by either the midwife or paediatrician.
- **In cases of fetal distress, there is an urgent need to get the baby out and to the infant resuscitaire. In this situation, the umbilical cord is really triple clamped using Kocher forceps or similar. The first clamp is applied further away from the base of the baby's umbilicus. The second clamp is then placed approximately 10 cm along and the cord cut – an umbilical vessel can be accessed if necessary as part of resuscitation measures. The infant is passed from the operating table. A third clamp is applied to the umbilicus, to allow the taking of cord blood for a blood gas analysis.**
- After delivery of the baby, the placenta is delivered by controlled cord traction.
- Sometimes the placental membranes can become slightly adherent to the uterine wall.

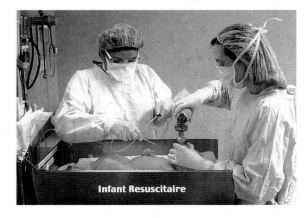

Fig. 11.5 Infant resuscitaire

- To ensure uterine haemostasis, it is essential that all membranous and placental tissue be removed from the uterine cavity. If the membranes do not fall away easily with the placenta, they are gently drawn off the uterine wall in a seesaw motion, using either Kocher forceps or Rampley sponge-holding forceps.
- Following delivery of the placenta, IV Syntocinon 10 units is given to the mother by the anaesthetist. This stimulates the uterus to contract and in doing so assists in controlling uterine blood loss and maintaining haemostasis.
- Uterine cavity is swabbed by the surgeon using a large sponge to exclude residual placental tissue or membrane. **If this is not done thoroughly and products are retained, there is the potential for postoperative complications including haemorrhage and/or infection.**
- Once this has been excluded, repair of the uterus can begin.
- To control bleeding and realign the opened uterine edges, Green Armytage clamps are used. They are applied to the incised edges of the uterus and/or to the mid-portion edges of the upper and lower incision line.
- Two-layer closure of the uterine incision is the most common. An absorbable suture, such as 1/0 Surgigut, is used as a continuous stitch.
- Once the uterus has been closed and haemostasis examined, the uterine fundus is massaged to firm.
- Pericolic gutters are swabbed of retained blood and amniotic fluid.
- Pelvic anatomy including the fallopian tubes, ovaries and uterus is checked to exclude any abnormality or possible pathology such as endometriosis, ovarian cysts or fibroid formation.
- It should be noted that while no longer routinely done, some obstetric surgeons will close the uterine peritoneum to secure possible bleeding from the edges of the visceral peritoneum. If this is done, 2/0 Surgigut or similar will be used.
- Once haemostasis is established and the uterus well contracted and firm, the rectus sheath can be closed. This is usually done using a monofilament absorbable suture such as a 1/0 Blosyn/Vicryl or Polysorb or equivalent.
- If required, a wound-drainage system such as a redivac drain will be positioned before closure of

the sheath. A drain can be considered in cases of prolonged labour or when the uterine incision has been closed in one layer only.

- On closure of the rectus sheath, some surgeons may choose to approximate the subcutaneous fat layer with several interrupted absorbable stitches. This is not routine but may be a surgeon's preference or done where additional support is required – such as in the obese patient. A plaingut or similar absorbable stitch will be used.
- Skin closure will be achieved using an absorbable subcuticular continuous stitch, such as 3/0 Vicryl. If the woman is obese, it is beneficial to apply interrupted tension stitches. Stitches are then removed between days 5 and 7 postoperation.
- Although more costly, staples are also frequently used for skin closure post-C/S. Cosmetically, research suggests a better result and fewer complications such as wound dehiscence and infection.
- Following wound closure, the area is cleaned and, according to surgeon preference, a dressing applied.
- It is routine for some surgeons to massage the uterine fundus again at the completion of the operation to expel any clots vaginally.
- Per rectum paracetamol and diclofenac suppositories (unless contraindicated) may be ordered by the anaesthetist and given at this point.
- When the anaesthetist is satisfied that all observations are stable, the woman can be moved from the operating table onto the postoperative bed and transferred to the Post-Anaesthesia Care Unit (PACU).

RECOVERY OF THE WOMAN POST-C/S

Hospital policy will dictate whether a midwife or a PACU nurse will attend to care in recovery. However, the same principles and standards apply. Depending on policy, the baby may or may not transfer into the recovery area with the mother. Ideally, if all has gone well at delivery for both parties, it is beneficial practice to promote bonding through early contact between the mother and her newborn. Where possible and if applicable, the father will also participate in and enjoy this experience. If the mother chooses to breastfeed her child, this can begin in the recovery room usually within the first hour of life.

C/S may be performed under any of the following anaesthetics.

- Epidural.
- Spinal.
- Combination of spinal and epidural.
  or
- GA.

The following considerations should be observed.

- Recovery of the woman should be in a well-lit environment in order for the staff to adequately observe vital signs and other observations, and to detect changes in these.
- For women who have undergone C/S under any of the above anaesthetic types, a minimum stay of 1 hour within a PACU is the norm.
- Nurse or midwife caring for the woman remains with her for the duration of this time. If he/she is relieved of these duties, a full handover of labour history, surgery and anaesthetic administration is required.
- Many PACUs do not permit support persons to remain with the woman. However, in the obstetric environment, this will depend entirely on the specific hospital and protocols followed. In some centres, it is not unusual for a support person (usually the father of the newborn) to accompany the woman and baby into the recovery room following an uncomplicated C/S. Other family members can visit the woman on the postnatal ward after discharge from the PACU.

Handover provided by the anaesthetist will include the following.

- Brief history of events leading to the OR.
- Operative procedure performed.
- Anaesthetic type.
- Drugs received to date – including pain relief in labour/pre-/intra- and postoperative medications.
- Estimated blood loss before and during surgery.
- Volume of IV fluids received pre-/intra- and postoperatively including labour.
- Vital sign recordings intraoperatively.
- Additional events or complications experienced throughout anaesthesia surgery.
- Postoperative fluid orders.
- Urine output.

Procedures conducted within the obstetric operating theatre environment

The following specific instructions are clarified.

- Removal of the epidural catheter.
- Further pain relief.
- Contact details for the anaesthetist from that point.
- Handover from the theatre midwife or nursing staff.

Postoperative observations following C/S

On arrival in the PACU and following handover from the anaesthetist and midwife, the following observations are recorded.

- Level of consciousness.
- Airway status.
- Blood pressure.
- Pulse.
- Respirations.
- Oxygen saturation.
- Block height – where an epidural or spinal block has been used.
- Wound site.
- Urine output: colour and volume noted on arrival to recovery. If the blood is stained, bladder trauma may have occurred during surgery.

The frequency of observation requirements will be dictated by the anaesthetist or by established standards and policies at each hospital facility. As a guide, the above observations are recorded as often as 5 minutes for the first 15 minutes and then every 15 minutes after that unless otherwise indicated.

When observations are stable, and if the mother wishes to, the baby may be offered a breastfeed. The person looking after the woman should be present at all times in the recovery period. Depending on the practice standards at any given facility, it is usual that the woman remain nil by mouth until she reports passing flatus. Following an uneventful recovery and having met all discharge criteria, the woman and baby can be transferred to the postnatal area.

Unless an epidural infusion has been ordered, the epidural catheter is removed before transfer from the PACU. The catheter tip must be sighted on removal and the site sprayed with spray dressing or a sterile dressing applied.

POSTNATAL HOSPITAL STAY FOLLOWING C/S – MOTHER

The usual length of stay post-C/S is 3–5 days but it depends greatly on the needs of the woman. The following factors are considered and met before discharge.

Satisfactory postoperative recovery period

- Vital signs in the first 24 hours are within normal parameters and have remained stable.
- Indwelling urinary catheter and IV therapy have been removed – usually the day following surgery. The woman has passed urine since this time.
- Vaginal bleeding has been within normal limits since delivery.
- Wound site is clean and dry – no signs of infection evident.
- Woman is mobilising freely. A physiotherapist will have seen the woman in the first day or two postsurgery and again before discharge. The physiotherapist offers instruction on deep breathing/gentle exercise and specific exercises to undertake post-C/S.
- Pain relief is under control.
- Woman's haemoglobin level is within acceptable parameters. It is checked on day 2 post-C/S.

Postnatal recovery period

The adjustment to the role of motherhood (particularly for first-time mothers) can be overwhelming during the first few months and especially in those early days. The following must be considered.

- Physiological changes within normal parameters: uterus involution, condition of the breasts and nipples, oedema to lower extremities, etc.
- Establishing confidence in mothercraft skills including breastfeeding/artificial feeding/nappy care and bathing can take some time.
- The woman may not feel ready to leave hospital if lacking confidence in these areas and should be encouraged to stay if this is the case.
- In some countries early discharge (24 hrs) is normal following a vaginal birth. After C/S however, discharge is more likely to be around the 5th post-operative day

- Psychological/emotional status: 'the blues' is a familiar term applied to new mothers around days 3–5 postnatally. Tearfulness for no apparent reason is common. This is usually put down to changing hormone levels and, interestingly, seems to coincide with breast engorgement associated with the establishment of the milk supply.
- Social factors: the home environment should be considered to establish what support the woman will have at home and if additional help is required. A social worker may provide assistance.
- Contraception is discussed by the medical practitioner or other health professional.
- Diet/wound care and signs of potential complications are also discussed before discharge.
- All women are followed up by their doctor or midwife in the postnatal period postdischarge. If there are any ongoing concerns, they can be identified or followed up at this time.
- Frequency of care will be dictated by need and the healthcare services offered in particular regions or country. Follow-up care may be more frequent for women post-C/S. In some countries, such as New Zealand, the woman is seen by her midwife within the first 24–48 hours of discharge and then daily or every second day as required.
- If all is well, care of both the mother and baby is handed over to the community nurse (Plunket nurse in New Zealand) at approximately 4 weeks. The obstetrician or general practitioner does the 6-week check.

THE BABY

It is usual practice for a midwife to be present at all deliveries including delivery by C/S. The midwife who provided theatre care for the woman will need to hand over additional information about labour history, and details on the baby.

- Time and date of birth.
- Sex of baby.
- Weight of baby.
- APGAR score.
- Drug administration.
- **It is essential that identification bracelets of both the mother and child are checked between staff members involved in care.**

ROUTINE MEASURE WHEN RECEIVING AND OBSERVING THE INFANT IN THE FIRST MINUTES OF LIFE (APPLIES FOR ALL DELIVERY METHODS)

- Baby is dried of blood and fluids using warm towels. Drying of hair and maintaining of body temperature is vital to infant wellbeing as heat loss can occur rapidly in the newborn. The process of drying provides gentle stimulation.
- Gentle suctioning of the oropharynx of blood or other fluids.
- Facial oxygen.

Table 11.9
APGAR score

The APGAR score is a numerical scoring system applied at 1 and 5 minutes of birth as a guide to evaluate the condition and status of the baby. Five observations are assessed:

1. Heart rate
2. Respiration
3. Muscle tone
4. Reflexes
5. Colour

- Two points are allocated for each of the five observations to give a total of 10 points
- Points are subtracted accordingly
- The first score is assessed at 1 minute of life, the second at 5 minutes and again at 10 minutes of life if required
- An APGAR score of 9 or 10 at 1 minute of life is usually achieved by the healthy term infant. A point may have been lost for colour or muscle tone. At 5 minutes, either of these observations may have improved so the baby then achieves an APGAR score of 10 at 5 minutes. In this case, the infant demonstrates a good heart rate, colour, muscle tone and reflexes, and breathing is well established.

- Further stimulation provided by the injection of vitamin K to a well baby will provoke a positive response: vigorous crying, muscle flexion and extension.
- The lower the APGAR score, the less ideal the condition of the baby. The initiation of resuscitation measures will apply according to the clinical assessment.
- In the majority of cases where the APGAR score is lower at 1 minute, the above measures are usually enough to prompt a favourable response and the baby will establish breathing and maintain an appropriate heart rate. An increase in the score at 5 minutes is reflective of this.

In other cases, further resuscitative measures are required to achieve a good outcome for the baby.

- Bag and mask ventilation.
- Aspiration of the airways via suction: use of a laryngoscope provides better vision if this is necessary – in some cases a meconium aspirator is required.
- Intubation.
- Insertion of an umbilical catheter and administration of resuscitative drugs.
- Cardiac massage.

Vitamin K

In most developed countries, babies are offered either oral or intramuscular vitamin K at birth. This is offered as a prophylactic measure to protect against haemorrhage in the newborn, which can occur due to a deficiency of vitamin K_1. Vitamin K is necessary for the formation of prothrombin. As the neonatal liver further matures, the baby will develop his/her own clotting factors. The risk of haemorrhage in the newborn increases in cases of traumatic delivery and/or instrumental delivery.

POSTNATAL CARE OF THE BABY BEFORE DISCHARGE

Following delivery post-C/S, the baby is thoroughly examined by the midwife or paediatrician.

- Well newborn can be transferred to the postnatal area with his/her mother.

- In most centres, 'rooming in' is encouraged, however, this may vary in places.
- Woman will be supported in caring for her baby in the first few days postoperatively.
- A well baby will have passed both urine and meconium within the first 24 hours of birth.
- Baby will be alert and feeding well either by breast or with an artificial formula.
- Some hospital facilities record a discharge weight. Unless the baby weighed < 2500 g at birth and providing he/she is feeding well and output is satisfactory, there is little indication for this practice.
- Most babies will lose up to 10% of their birth weight in the first week of life. This is usually regained in the following 10 days.[1]
- If there are no specific medical or surgical conditions requiring treatment, the baby will be discharged home with the mother.

References

1. Olds SB, London ML, Ladewig PAW. *Maternal–Newborn Nursing: A Family and Community-based Approach*, 6th edn. Upper Saddle River: Prentice Hall Heath, 2000.
2. Beischer NA, Mackay EV, Colditz PB. *Obstetrics and the Newborn: An Illustrated Text Book*, 3rd edn. London: WB Saunders, 1999.
3. Zanetta G, Tampieri A, Currado I, Regalia A, Nespoli A, Midwife T, Fei F, Colombo C, Bottino S. Changes in Cesarean delivery in an Italian university hospital, 1982–1996: a comparison with the national trend. *Birth* 1999; 26: 144–148.
4. Shearer EL. Cesarean section: medical benefits and costs. *Soc Sci Med* 1993; 37: 1223–1231.
5. Walsh D. Electronic fetal heart monitoring: revisited and reappraised. *Br J Midwife* 1998; 6: 400–404.
6. Gregory KD, Curtin SC, Taffel SM, Notzon FC. Changes in indications for Cesarean delivery: United States, 1985 and 1994. *Am J Public Health* 1998; 88: 1384–1387.
7. Poma PA. Rupture of a Cesarean-scarred uterus: a community hospital experience. *J Natl Med Assoc* 2000; 92: 295–300.
8. Shimonovitz S, Botosneano A, Hochner-Celnikier D. Successful first vaginal birth after Cesarean section: a predictor of reduced risk for uterine rupture in subsequent deliveries. *Isr Med Assoc J*. 2000; 2: 526–528.
9. Trueba G, Contreras C, Velazco MT, Garcia-Lara E, Martinez HB. Alternative strategy to decrease Cesarean section: support by Doulas during labor. *J Perinat Educ* 2000; 9: 8–13.

10. Goh J, Flynn M. *Examination Obstetrics and Gynaecology*. Sydney: MacLennan & Petty, 1996.

11. Kattan SA. Maternal urological injuries associated with vaginal deliveries: change of pattern. *Int Urol Nephrol* 1997; 29: 155–161.

12. James DK, Steer PJ, Weiner CP, Gonik B. *High Risk Pregnancy: Management Options*, 2nd edn. London: WB Saunders, 1999.

Procedures conducted within the obstetric operating theatre environment

Index